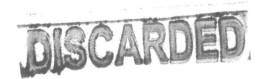

Stuttering

C. Woodruff Starkweather
Janet Givens-Ackerman

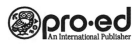
pro·ed
An International Publisher

8700 Shoal Creek Boulevard
Austin, Texas 78757-6897

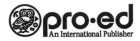

© 1997 by PRO-ED, Inc.
8700 Shoal Creek Boulevard
Austin, Texas 78757-6897

The PRO-ED **Studies in Communicative Disorders** series
Series Editor: Harvey Halpern

Library of Congress Cataloging-in-Publication Data

Starkweather, C. Woodruff.
    Stuttering / C. Woodruff Starkweather, Janet Givens-Ackerman.
      p.   cm.
    Includes bibliographical references and index.
    ISBN 0-89079-699-8 (pbk. : alk. paper)
    1. Stuttering.   I. Givens-Ackerman, Janet. II. Title.
RC424.S693   1997
616.85'54—dc20
                                               96-20276
                                                 CIP

This book is designed in Eras and Palatino.

Production Manager: Alan Grimes
Production Coordinator: Karen Swain
Managing Editor: Tracy Sergo
Designer: Thomas Barkley
Reprints Buyer: Alicia Woods
Editor: Lisa Tippett
Editorial Assistant: Claudette Landry
Editorial Assistant: Martin Wilson

Printed in the United States of America

2 3 4 5 6 7 8 9 10   00 99 98

People who stutter comprise about 1% of the adult population. To the countless numbers of them who have already begun their journey of self-discovery, we would like to dedicate this book.

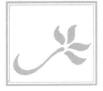

Contents

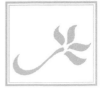

Preface

Much has happened since the first volume on stuttering in the PRO-ED Series on Communicative Disorders was published in 1986. There are electronic (e-)mail discussion lists between professional speech clinicians and people who stutter on the Internet, an active Special Interest Division in Fluency within the American Speech and Hearing Association (ASHA), and the likelihood that specialty recognition in stuttering treatment will soon be a reality. There are also changes in the political climate that will have an effect on stuttering. Perhaps most important, new and promising methods of treatment are being developed.

We introduce such an approach in this book. Still in the developmental stage, it consists of a number of approaches and ideas that have been helpful for many thousands of people in working on other kinds of problems. It seems reasonable that these approaches hold promise for alleviating aspects of the stuttering problem that have not been adequately dealt with in the past, and we have founded the Birch Tree Foundation upon these principles.

It has been said that speech pathologists have the information (and therefore the understanding) about stuttering that must be the basis of any treatment but they lack the tools, whereas psychologists have the tools but lack the information (and therefore the understanding). This book is an attempt to give speech pathologists some additional tools—ones that have proven their usefulness for working on similar problems.

The book, however, is not just for speech pathologists. It is written also for people who stutter, their friends and family, and the parents of children who stutter. In today's world, there is a recognition of the necessity and importance of including the client, or the client's parents, in the process of evaluation and treatment. The new approach to treatment we describe is based on the idea that the client (or parent) and clinician (or supportive partner) together can deal with stuttering far more effectively than either can alone. It is for this reason that the book is co-authored by a person who stutters. Our collaboration exemplifies one aspect of this new way of looking at the treatment of stuttering.

Acknowledgments

I would like to acknowledge my gratitude to a number of people. They may not have been specifically involved with this book, but their influence on me is unmistakable. First, I am very grateful for the opportunity to work with Janet. Her ideas, writing skill, and editorial ability are woven into the fabric of this book so that it can reach those who stutter, their families, and their friends. I am also grateful to the clients I have seen over the past 26 years and to my correspondents on the Internet. They have taught me far more about the disorder than any textbook. I have also learned a great deal from my students, particularly Joy Armson, Barbara Amster, and Meryl Wall. My gratitude to my teachers, formal and informal, is inexpressible. I have learned from Stan Ainsworth, Oliver Bloodstein, Dick Boehmler, Gene Brutten, Paul Czuchna, Hugo Gregory, the late Hal Luper, Al Murphy, Joe Sheehan, Hal Starbuck, the late Charles Van Riper, and the late Dean Williams. I appreciate also insightful discussion with (or lectures from) my contemporaries: Gordon Blood, the late Einer Boberg, Ed Conture, Dick Curlee, Luc De Nil, Marie-Christine Franken, Sheryl Gottwald, Barry Guitar, Murray Halfond, Diane Hill, Wouter Hulstijn, Pascal van Lieshout, Christy Ludlow, Catherine Montgomery, Megan Neilson, Herman Peters, Peter Ramig, Phil Schneider, Anne Smith, Ken St. Louis, and Janice Westbrook. I am grateful, too, for the support and friendship I have received from many members of the National Stuttering Project, especially John Ahlbach, Annie Bradberry, Judith Eckardt, Michael Sugarman, and Paul Young.

C. Woodruff Starkweather

I have believed from the beginning that this book would provide me with an opportunity to have an impact on a profession that did not serve me very well when I needed it most. The speech therapists I was sent to in grade school were ignorant at best and controlling and manipulative at worst. It is for that reason that I wanted so much for this book to be accessible to those outside the profession—to people who want to know more about this disorder and how they can help, whether they are family, friends, or people who themselves stutter. What impact this book will have remains to be seen. I am, first of all, thankful to Woody for making this opportunity possible.

I wish to also thank the following people for the impact they have had on my life: Melodie Beatty, whose writings not only inspired me but provided a solid foundation for my early recovery work and who first exposed me to the simplicity of the awareness-acceptance-change model; my anonymous friends in various 12-step recovery programs who teach me, through their example, one day at a time, how important it is to "keep the focus on myself"; my professional guides along this journey I'm on: Anne Cook Finnegan, Nell Taylor, and Brian Gill; and the facilitators at the Gestalt Institute of Cleveland. Each of these people offered me a room safe and warm enough that I could remove my protective cloak of denial and begin to truly look at myself. Finally, a special word of thanks to my two sons, Jonathan and David, who remind me, as nothing else can, of all the things I cannot change—and how that's OK.

Janet Givens-Ackerman

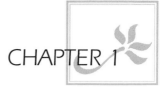
Introduction

S tuttering is a devastating disorder that afflicts about 1% of the world's population at any given time. The probability of a person ever stuttering during his or her lifetime is about 5%. Unlike most other speech and language disorders, stuttering takes over a person's life. It dominates one's sense of identity and makes every sentence a minefield of frustration, humiliation, and shame. Although the specific cause of this problem is not yet known, and no easy solutions are available for adults who stutter, there are effective treatments that can lead to a dramatic reduction in the symptoms. The burden can be laid down, and the person can discover the possibility of a normal life.

Charles Van Riper, an early pioneer in the field of treatment for stuttering who had a severe stutter, often said that his life began at the age of 30, when he discovered that he could stutter in a much easier way. His childhood, youth, and early adulthood were a wasteland of misery. Thereafter, he dedicated his life to finding solutions and solving the riddle of stuttering. All speech clinicians and researchers in the area of fluency have taken up this challenge. Few areas of speech and language pathology provide the excitement and satisfaction for clinicians and the thrill of discovery for researchers that the fluency area does.

Historical Perspective

Changes in Understanding

In the past 10 years, since the first book in the PRO-ED Studies in Communicative Disorders series was published, major gains in the understanding of stuttering have been made through research and insight. We have learned much about the way in which the speech mechanism moves in the process of producing speech sounds, and this information has been coupled with a clearer understanding of the rather different movements that people who stutter make. We have come to understand far more clearly than before some of the mysteries of stuttering, such as its tendency to be absent when the person who stutters reads in chorus with another person or speaks slowly or under altered feedback. We have reached a better understanding of how stuttering develops, of the role of the family in the process of development, and of the role of learning processes. Through research, we have also been able to set aside certain theoretical ideas—that stuttering is simply a voice problem or that it is only a language problem—and this has cleared the way for more focused research.

Changes in Therapy

At the same time, we have developed a number of new assessment and therapy techniques, and we have reached consensus on a number of therapeutic issues that severely divided the field in the past. During the 1970s and 1980s, clinicians tried to (a) shape the client's stuttering into normal nonfluency, or (b) shape the client's speech into perfect fluency. These two approaches rested on different assumptions and differed in the type of outcome they produced. Both approaches had their shortcomings. In the debate that this division produced, there was often more heat than light; however, 10 to 20 years later, things have changed. In a recent survey (Starkweather, 1994), nearly all clinicians combined these two approaches into a new way of seeing the problem and a new, more "eclectic," way of treating it.

There has also been a major change in the way speech clinicians deal with the very young person who stutters. No longer do we wait to see if preschool children will "outgrow" the problem,[1] because we have learned that by waiting we condemn a significant proportion of these children to a childhood filled with shame and embarrassment, low self-esteem, and failure. In addition, we have discovered that treating the very young child is not only highly successful, but also

---

[1]There have always been a number of speech clinicians and pediatricians who do not adopt the "wait-and-see" attitude. Both speech clinicians and pediatricians are changing in this regard, although, sad to say, the advice is still given by some individuals.

remarkably easy, and that it does not contain some of the drawbacks common in adult treatment.

Political Changes

The Self-Help Movement

Changes have also occurred in the political climate. During the 1980s and early 1990s self-help groups became much larger and more powerful (Ramig, 1993). Their appeal to people who stutter rests on the fact that the pain that these people feel can be alleviated through the support of others with the same problem. When people who stutter talk to each other, they do not feel the judgment and criticism that they feel when talking in the everyday world; instead, they feel an atmosphere of acceptance. The point is that, in an atmosphere where they do not feel such a strong need to struggle with their stuttering, they can "let it go." When they do this, the stuttering itself is often powerfully alleviated. Theorists need to be aware of this force, and clinicians need to make use of it. The newest approach to stuttering treatment combines the powerful forces of the self-help movement, selected psychological therapies, and elements of tried-and-true speech therapy techniques.

A very modern form of the self-help movement can be found on the Internet, where currently there are at least two discussion groups on stuttering—STUTT-L and STUT-HLP.[2] The STUTT-L list includes clinicians and researchers, as well as people who stutter, in a wide variety of dialogue about stuttering. Information about stuttering and for those who stutter can be found at a Gopher site and a World Wide Web site.[3]

The STUTT-L list began as a way for researchers and clinicians to share their experiences in trying to understand stuttering, but it was soon joined by people who stuttered who wanted to find out about the latest research and treatments. It evolved into an academically flavored "electronic self-help group" (Starkweather, 1995a). The support and insights gained through these discussion groups have been

---

[2]To join STUTT-L, send a message to LISTSERV@VM.TEMPLE.EDU that says SUB STUTT-L Yourfirstname Yourlastname. To join STUT-HLP, send a message to LIST-PROC2@BGU.EDU that says SUB STUT-HLP Yourfirstname Yourlastname.

[3]The Gopher site can be accessed at gopher.mankato.msus.edu. To send materials to the Gopher site, address them to Judy Kuster at KUSTER@VAX1.MANKATO.MSUS.EDU. The World Wide Web site may be accessed through http://hermes.bioc.uvic.ca.

very helpful to many individuals and, in a few cases, have been vitally instrumental in someone's recovery.

The Role of Discrimination

Along with the increased empowerment that self-help groups and Internet lists have given to their members, there has been an increased awareness of discrimination. Discrimination against people who stutter is widespread. The cruelty of schoolchildren and the jokes and mimicry of adolescents have become institutionalized in frequent media depictions of stuttering as something to laugh about. From Porky Pig to *A Fish Called Wanda*, screenwriters and stand-up comics have made fun of the struggles of people who stutter. Fifty years ago, it would have been common to see the struggles of a person with cerebral palsy or the mistakes of an individual with mental retardation similarly caricatured for the sake of comedy. It is hoped that we soon will be past the point where people who stutter are the objects of comedy. The National Stuttering Project (NSP)[4] has won some impressive battles against the media, and the continued work of the NSP and the Stuttering Foundation of America (SFA)[5] in educating the public about this disorder have made substantial gains in reducing discrimination.

It is a different story in the workplace. Discrimination against people who stutter has been well documented and is widespread (Hurst & Cooper, 1983). It can occur in the hiring, promotion, or even the firing of individuals. Part of a larger form of discrimination based on speech, discrimination against people who stutter is probably the worst part of the problem. The Americans with Disabilities Act of 1990 (ADA) defines a disability as any characteristic, or perceived characteristic, that interferes with the performance of a major life activity. These activities are listed in the ADA, and speech is one of them. Because stuttering quite clearly interferes with speech, it is without doubt a disability in the legal sense. Discrimination in the workplace

---

[4]The NSP, a membership organization for people who stutter, has over 60 self-help chapters throughout the United States. It is the largest such organization in the world. See Appendix C for the address of the NSP and other worldwide resources for people who stutter.

[5]The SFA (formerly the Speech Foundation of America) is perhaps the oldest nonprofit organization dedicated to the prevention and treatment of stuttering. Founded by businessman Malcolm Fraser in 1947, it publishes high-quality books and pamphlets and other information to educate the public about stuttering. In addition, it sponsors training programs for specialists in stuttering treatment, produces films, and operates a very busy telephone information service (800/967-7700).

that is based on disability is against the law. A few suits have been brought against employers for discriminating in the hiring, firing, or promotion of people who stutter. Although no case law has yet been written, these cases have been settled in a way that makes it evident that the ADA can be used to achieve either compliance with the law in hiring and promotion or redress for firing in a discriminatory way.

People who stutter can perform a wide variety of job tasks, usually more than they believe they can. Their use of language in written form is often exquisitely articulate (e.g., Ahlbach, 1995), a fact that has often been demonstrated on the Internet. When people who stutter use spoken language, it may take them a little longer[6] to communicate, but this should not be seen as different from the wheelchair-bound person who can perform most tasks even though it may take him or her a little longer to get around. It is unreasonable to deny a person who stutters a position on the grounds that her or his stuttering may slow performance to a small degree. In the same way, a person's stuttering should not disqualify him or her from performing a job where, for example, the image of the company is at stake (such as answering the telephone), any more than a person in a wheelchair should be denied a receptionist's position because it might negatively influence the company's image.

The ADA requires that employer's make a "reasonable accommodation" to anyone with a disability who is employed by the company. A reasonable accommodation might be having someone else answer the telephone, if that is particularly difficult for the person who stutters. One individual who sued his employer after being fired because of his stuttering argued successfully that the supervisor could reasonably have adopted a less rude and overbearing style of management when talking to him. Employers are also required to make such accommodations as purchasing a fluency-enhancing device or paying for speech therapy for the employee who stutters. Many employers will do these things without being compelled; however, not all will do so, and the law thus is a valuable aid in helping the person who stutters (a) gain access to work for which he or she is otherwise qualified, (b) seek promotion to a level commensurate with his or her skill, and (c) retain a job when performance has been satisfactory.

---

[6]On the average, stuttering behaviors add only a minute quantity of time to the performance of a job, although it may seem very long to co-workers who at first are not used to the delays stuttering presents.

The Reduction in Training Standards

A third important change in the political climate was brought about by the American Speech-Language-Hearing Association (ASHA).[7] In 1993, the standards of training were revised by the Council on Professional Standards (COPS). The primary responsibility of COPS is protecting the public served by the certified members of ASHA, specifically, to verify that the level of training speech pathologists receive is adequate to ensure a competent performance of the common practices of speech therapy. The revisions made in 1993 weakened this protection. Whereas in former years a specific number of hours of training was required for each of the basic speech disorders—stuttering, articulation disorder, and voice disorder—the new standards required hours only for "speech disorders," without specifying how many hours needed to be obtained for each disorder. The change was implemented so that the training programs could have, in the words of the council, "more flexibility" in meeting ASHA standards. In practice, it meant that programs could cut back on their training of students in the areas where clients are difficult to find—stuttering and voice disorders. A survey conducted only a year after the new standards were put into effect (Starkweather & Bishop, 1994) found that two thirds of the surveyed programs had cut back on either the required academic coursework or the clinical practicum in the area of stuttering.

It is important to note that this change, which exposed people who stutter to an increased probability of receiving therapy from poorly trained clinicians, was made without consulting any of the groups that represent people who stutter. It was implemented without informing the public or asking for their opinion. For these reasons, in the opinion of many individuals, the change was an unethical act[8], and it enraged clinicians. The Certificate of Clinical Competence (CCC),[9] which had always been the standard of preparation in speech pathology, had been degraded.

---

[7]ASHA is a professional association of speech–language pathologists and audiologists. See Appendix C for its address.

[8]ASHA's Code of Ethics states as its first principle that "Individuals shall honor their responsibility to hold paramount the welfare of persons they serve professionally."

[9]The Certificate of Clinical Competence is a credential granted by ASHA attesting that the holder of the certificate has followed a course of study that meets certain specified minimal standards of preparation for the practice of speech–language pathology (CCC-S) or audiology (CCC-A).

These changes have come very close to legalizing the practice of charlatanism, that is, giving people credentials that the public believes qualify them to treat stuttering when, in fact, they are not so qualified. Only a weak line in ASHA's Code of Ethics, which tells clinicians they should not practice in areas for which they are not qualified, protects the public from untrained practitioners.

Several good consequences came out of this debacle. First was a movement to establish a form of *specialty recognition* that gained force and moved quickly to a successful conclusion. By the time this book is in print, a process will be in place to acknowledge clinicians who are especially well prepared to treat people who stutter. This change has long been needed in the field, and it will be very helpful in ensuring that people who stutter will receive treatment that is up to standard.

A second good consequence of the weakening of standards has been an *increase in the political awareness* of the clinicians who serve people who stutter. This increased politicization of an important segment of the field will surely benefit people who stutter in the long run. Several organizations became much stronger as a result of this change in awareness, for example, the International Fluency Association and ASHA's Special Interest Division on Fluency.

A third good consequence of the reduced standards was the development of *Guidelines for the Practice of Stuttering Treatment* (Starkweather, Blood, St. Louis, Peters, & Westbrook, 1995). These guidelines, developed by the Special Interest Division on Fluency, are reprinted in their entirety in Appendix A of this book. They describe a set of agreed-upon goals for stuttering treatment, procedures that are known to be effective in reaching those goals, and the competencies that clinicians will need in order to carry out those procedures. As a result, any clinician can compare his or her skills against the guidelines to determine if further education might be useful in particular areas. People who stutter may compare the training of the clinicians they may want to use against the guidelines to see if they are current on practices that are being employed.

Although not all of these changes are good ones, they are part of the climate in which research on stuttering and treatment of this very problematic disorder are currently taking place. With an increased awareness of this current climate, it is hoped that clients, clinicians, parents, and friends can work together to help the person who stutters achieve a successful recovery from stuttering in the most effective manner.

The Politics of Terminology

The Word "Stutterer"

Many people who stutter resent being called stutterers. They believe that the label *stutterer* characterizes them as a disorder first and as a person second. These individuals prefer to be called a "person who stutters" to make it clear that they are individuals first and people who stutter second. At the same time, others who stutter believe that the term "person who stutters" (or PWS, as it is often shortened) is a kind of euphemism—a softening of the harsh reality of the disorder and, as such, a form of avoidance that does not serve the person well.

Stuttering has an impact on a person's sense of self to varying degrees. Language can be a window through which the clinician can model an attitude toward the disorder that is nonavoidant and unafraid. Unfortunately, many clinicians *are* afraid of the disorder and even of the word that labels it. They choose to call stuttering "having difficulty" or "getting into trouble," which tells the client that his or her fear and avoidance must be justified if even a speech clinician is afraid to utter the evil "S" word.

Listening to the way clients describe themselves is instructional (e.g., I am a stutterer, I have a stutter, I stutter). The impact of language on identity (and vice versa) is one of many areas in need of further research.

Speech clinicians need to raise the topic of terminology early in their conversations with their clients. It would be unfortunate to use the word stutterer when talking to someone who was offended by it; yet, it is always therapeutically useful to be as straightforward as possible. Communication between the clinician and client is the best way to clear up any misunderstanding that may arise as a result of the use of one term over another.

St. Louis and Sielen (1994a, b) looked at the public's view of these terms, comparing the "person-first" with "non–person-first" term for a variety of different disorders and conditions. In addition, they assessed the level of stigmatization for the terms about which they asked. Interestingly, the public showed very little preference. The person-first and the non–person-first terms were considered about equal in preference. This was equally true for the pair *stutterer* versus *person who stutters*. Only those terms with a high level of stigmatization, such as psychotic and leper, met with strong disapproval. The term stutterer, it turned out, did not have a high degree of stigmatization attached to it.

Impairment, Disability, and Handicap

Another distinction is also useful. We can speak first of stuttering as an *impairment*, something that is wrong with the syllables and words a person produces. All people who stutter are impaired in this sense. Second, this impairment can interfere with the process of communication by taking up speech time without contributing information and by calling unwanted attention to the way in which words are spoken, thus distracting the listener from the content. To the extent that these two things occur, stuttering is a *disability*. The extent of the disability can be measured by the percentage of speaking time that stuttering behaviors occupy and by the extent to which the presence of these behaviors distract listeners. Beyond this level, a person who stutters may find that the presence of the disorder interferes with his or her life in significant ways. To the extent that it does so, stuttering is a *handicap*. The person who stutters may be unwilling to initiate social contacts, apply for jobs where he or she feels speech is important, or use the telephone. To the extent that the person's life is disrupted, stuttering is a handicapping condition (Prins, 1991).

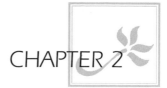

CHAPTER 2

Definition of Terms

A s in any specialization, there are specific terms, used by both the professional and by the individuals who suffer from the disorder, that make it easier to communicate about the problem and its characteristics. In this chapter, these terms will be defined so that a more common language can be used. Since the time of the Socratic dialogues, definitions have been the means by which any search for understanding can begin; therefore, these definitions are offered in the hope that they may make possible the first step toward better understanding.

Fluency

Once used to refer simply to the absence of stuttering, the term *fluency* has more usefully been viewed since the mid-1980s as referring to a skill possessed by all people in varying degrees. What is meant here is not language fluency—the ability to speak a language with minimal effort in finding words, constructing grammatical sentences, or pronunciation—but instead *speech* fluency: fluency of speech production. The word fluency comes from a Latin word that means flowing along, like a stream. Inherent in the meaning of this word are the twin concepts of movement and smoothness.

Consequently, speech fluency consists of two related variables—*continuity* and *rate*. The continuity of speech is the smoothness with which it is produced. If a person says, "I, *well, I went to the, uh, I mean I* went to the game," we recognize quickly that the italicized words are extraneous to the speaker's intention. The intended utterance, which is easy to discern for native speakers of the language, is "I went to the game." The extraneous parts are discontinuous; they break up the smooth flow of the intended sentence.

Normal Discontinuities

Types

There are many forms of normal discontinuity, but four main types are commonly recognized in regular speech: repetitions, pauses, false starts, and parenthetical remarks (Kowal, O'Connell, & Sabin, 1975).

Repetitions, as in the extraneous *"I went to the"* in the previous example, are probably the most noticeable type. The unit that is repeated may be as long as a phrase, as in the example, or it may be shorter, as in whole-word repetitions" *("I, I* went to the game"), or even a part of a word (I went to the g-game). Repetitions may also vary in their duration. The sentence "I, I, I, I, *went to the, went to the,* went to the game" contains two repetitions. The first is a whole-word repetition that is three units in length (note that one of the "I"s is part of the intended utterance and is consequently not counted as extraneous speech behavior) and one phrase repetition that is two units in length.

Repetitions are relatively rare in the speech of nonstutterers; when they do occur they are quite brief, usually only one iteration, and they are more likely to contain longer units of speech production, such as a phrase or a word. In the speech of people who stutter, by contrast, repetitions are more frequent, longer, and more likely to contain shorter units of speech production (e.g., "I *w-w-w-w-w*-went to the *g-g-g*-game").

The second type of normal discontinuity is the *pause,* which has two subtypes—filled and unfilled. The *unfilled pause* is simply a period of silence in the ongoing stream of speech that is recognizable as being extraneous to the utterance. Some pauses are an aspect of speech rhythm reflecting sentence structure (Bedore & Leonard, 1995; Van Lancker, Canter, & Terbeek, 1981). Such pauses tend to be shorter, and, by convention, pauses shorter than 250 msec are considered not to be extraneous to the intended utterance (Kowal et al., 1975). Unfilled pauses distributed with regard to sentence structure occur most frequently at clause boundaries. The pauses that occur within clauses seem more unusual and may be quite short, yet are still to be considered extraneous to the utterance. No specific protocol exists for distinguishing maximum duration of within-clause pauses. Therefore, if it is noticed, it is considered extraneous.

The *filled pause* is the sound "uh" or "um," which was described once, and most inaccurately, as "the sound of a mind going into neutral" (Perkins, 1971). Indeed, during the filled pause, the mind is quite actively planning what is to be said next, or searching for *le mot juste*. It is the mouth that is in neutral. In our culture and other similar cultures, the filled pause is in fact a kind of convention that signals to the speaker's interlocutor that the speaker has not finished his or her thought, as though there will be a brief pause due to technical difficulties (word finding, sentence construction, or a cognitive interruption such as "I am about to say something really stupid"). The pause is filled to retain the floor, that is, avoid interruption. Because the filled pause reveals the speaker as less than perfectly prepared to continue, it feels like an error in speech and is often treated as such, but, in fact, it is a useful conversational device.

Filled pauses tend to be longer than unfilled pauses, and it is a fair presumption that any pause that has lasted beyond a certain period of time, probably a little less than a full second, is likely to get filled with the "um" sound so as to avoid interruption.

In some Native American cultures, when a speaker before an audience hesitates for an appreciable period of time, the audience all produce a choral "uuuuuuuuh" until it is evident that the speaker is prepared to continue. This convention is simply a somewhat more polite version of the Anglo-European filled pause "uh." In Native American cultures, it is the audience that says "uh" to reassure the speaker that he or she still has the floor. The utility of either of these conventions is obvious. None of us is perfect, and on occasions any speaker needs a little extra time to formulate either the cognitive or the linguistic process of speaking.

The third kind of normal discontinuity is the *false start*. An example might be "*I went to the sh-*, I went to the game." The speaker, remembering that the halftime show was particularly entertaining, begins to say "I went to the show" but realizes that this is not appropriate for the intention, stops, and starts over again. Sometimes false starts cover impending social faux pas or logical or factual errors, such as "That dress is *awf-*, really interesting." Or "After the trial, Socrates drank the poisonous *wedl-*, I mean hemlock."

The fourth kind of normal discontinuity is the *parenthetical remark*, which is an interjected comment designed to appear as if it has the purpose of intensifying or refining the speaker's intention. In reality, its purpose is no different from that of the filled pause—to stall for time without losing the floor while the speaker thinks more completely of what he or she wants to say. Examples are the ubiquitous "I mean," "like," and "you know," as in "I mean, I mean, I want to go but, like, it isn't, you know, exactly my cup of tea, you know what I mean?" As children develop during the school years, there is a strong tendency for parenthetical remarks to replace the more childlike repetitions and the more socially undesirable "um." As a result, there is sometimes a large increase in parenthetical remarks during the teenage years, much to the consternation of many parents.

The overall level of continuity seems to change only minimally with growth. Yairi (1982) counted the number of discontinuities in normal 2-year-old children. He found that one third of these children in the earliest stages of acquiring the ability to produce sentences had speech that was no more discontinuous than that of an adult (1% to 2% discontinuously produced words). Another third had speech that was only slightly less continuous (3% to 4% discontinuously produced words) than that of adults. Only one third of the children in the sample had speech that was discontinuous enough to call attention to itself (>4%). Figure 2.1 provides the date from Yairi's study in a graphic format.

The Role of Formality

It is worth noting that the circumstances under which speech is occurring have a powerful effect on the noticeability of discontinuities. In the most formal circumstances where there is no audience interaction, such as a radio or TV broadcast, discontinuities are highly noticeable and distracting or annoying to the listening audience. In the next most formal circumstance—a live speech before an audience—discontinuities are slightly annoying and may be noticeable, which is why students who are bored with their instructor may start to count "ums." In the least formal circumstances—a one-to-one conversation where there is ample opportunity for interaction—"ums" and other forms of discontinuity are scarcely noticeable and often are not even recognized as having occurred (Goldman-Eisler, 1961).

The Role of Intention

When people who do not stutter speak, listeners infer the message that is intended (Levelt, 1989), in spite of the presence of a surprisingly

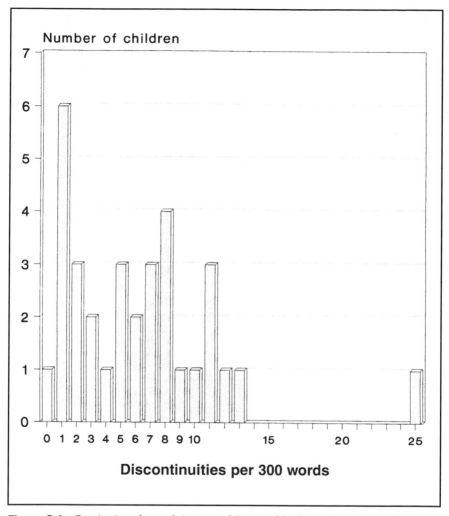

Figure 2.1. Continuity of speech in normal 2-year-olds. From "Longitudinal Studies of Disfluencies in Two-Year-Old Children," by E. Yairi, 1982, *Journal of Speech and Hearing Research, 25,* pp. 155–160.

large number of extraneous (not intentional) elements (Goldman-Eisler, 1961). Listeners pay little attention to aspects of the utterance that are not part of the intention, unless these extraneous elements are excessive or unusual in certain ways. Hegde and Hartman (1979a, 1979b) had subjects who were native speakers listen to tapes containing various quantities of normal discontinuities. They found that when single-unit, whole-word repetitions (usually a normal discontinuity) reached a frequency of 15% of the spoken words, they seemed to exceed a threshold level and were judged to be abnormal. And when "um" (also a normal type of discontinuity) reached a frequency of 20%, it also was judged to be abnormal. Unfortunately, similar information with regard to other types of discontinuities is lacking.

Measuring Continuity

When there are few or no extraneous elements, speech flows along, and the spoken message corresponds closely to the intended message. Under these circumstances, the utterance is "fluent" in one particular way: it has a high degree of continuity. Breaks in the flow of the intended message, or discontinuities, are composed of the extraneous elements mentioned above. The continuity of speech thus can be understood to be nothing more than the amount of correspondence between intention and utterance. This correspondence can be most directly assessed by measuring the amount of time taken up by all the extraneous portions of the utterance and dividing that amount by the total duration of the whole utterance, including both extraneous and intended portions. The result is the percentage of discontinuous speech time (PDST), which is a direct measure of the fluency of speech. This measure has the advantage of including both the frequency and the duration of discontinuous behaviors (See Chapter 5 for more discussion and a worked example).

Speech Rate

The rate of speech is the second element of fluency. Rate can be understood at two levels—the word and the syllable. At the word level, the measurement of *speech rate,* made with the discontinuities included, expresses the speed with which the person is able to make information flow. The average speech rate of normal male speakers in conversation is 167.7 words per minute (wpm), 220.6 syllables per minute (spm). Normal female speakers talk a little more slowly, at 151.2 wpm, 204.2 spm, and use longer words, but fewer ones, than do men (Lutz & Mallard, 1986).

At the syllable level, *articulatory rate,* with the discontinuities excluded, is assessed. This measure reflects the speed with which a person can move the structures of speech. Although not entirely free of influence from linguistic planning and sentence formulation, articulatory rate more closely measures speech motor control than speech rate does, because it is assumed that in normal speakers the discontinuities that are included in speech rate reflect linguistic planning. Articulatory rate depends upon two underlying variables—the velocity with which the parts of the vocal tract move and the extent to which adjacent movements overlap. The latter of these two aspects is known as *coarticulation*. For example, when saying the syllable /su/, the lips are rounded during the production of the /s/. It isn't necessary to wait until the /s/ is complete to begin rounding the lips for /u/, and this saves considerable time with minimal loss of intelligibility. As the rate of speech production increases, however, and coarticulatory overlap is increased, intelligibility begins to decline. Walker and Black (1950) found that normal speakers produce 5 to 6 syllables per second (300 to 600 spm).

The Relation Between Rate and Continuity

Continuity and rate are variables whose relationship can be expressed in two different ways. First, as a person talks more slowly, his or her utterance is likely to be more continuous. Second, the presence of discontinuities in an utterance slows the production of the intended message (Sheehan, 1970). If smoothness is desirable, it is sometimes possible with training to slow down and allow enough time for the linguistic and motor planning to occur during speech, thus removing the need for filled pauses and other forms of discontinuity. Television and radio broadcasters, who speak under the most formal of circumstances where there is no possibility of interaction with the audience, need to achieve speech that is free of discontinuities. They usually do so by learning to talk more slowly and, if they pause, to refrain from inserting filler sounds.

Speech Effort

Rate and continuity are the two visible manifestations of an underlying construct that seems to be at the heart of fluency. This construct is the ease, or effort, with which speech is produced (Starkweather, 1987). Fluent speakers are those who can produce long strings of syllables without apparent effort, as shown by their combination of rapid rate and continuous utterance. In other words, not only do they produce an utterance that matches their intention closely, but they are able to produce this match without slowing down, either by inserting pause time or by reducing the velocity of movement of the parts of the vocal tract.

Voluntariness and Automaticity

There seems to be little difference between people who stutter and people who don't with regard to the *voluntariness* of speech. The rapid, continuous production of syllables in normal speakers depends on the semiautomatic nature of speech production. Speech production is less voluntary than most other human behaviors. Most people who do not stutter produce words and syllables with less thought than they do such habitual behaviors as driving or swinging a tennis racket. There are, in fact, few behaviors that share the level of *automaticity* found in speech production. Even highly practiced musicians or skilled typists employ their particular skills with more thought than typical normal speakers do in ordinary talking. Ideally, speakers think, decide to make (some of) their thoughts public, construct the sentences, find the words, and string together the syllables with little or no additional thought. This characteristic of normal speech production has evolved, quite naturally, so that when we are talking our conscious minds are available to consider the ideas we wish to communicate or those we might be receiving from our listeners. It is quite inconceivable that we might have to talk for the purpose of communication while at the same time being responsible for each of the movements involved in speech production. The exact nature of the process by which the movements of speech are controlled in this semiautomatic way is currently a topic of intense investigation (Starkweather & Peters, 1995).

In addition, most speakers are also able to make a number of voluntary changes in their speech—adopting a different dialect, slowing down or speeding up, changing the pitch of the voice, choosing a different word, or constructing a sentence in another way. However, it is quite difficult for these voluntary alterations in output to be sustained for any length of time. Like breathing, speech production is thus highly automatic yet capable of being brought under voluntary control, at least temporarily. Many, probably most, individuals who stutter have exactly this same level of control with regard to word choice, dialect, vocal parameters, and so forth. Also, many of these individuals can (with considerable concentration) speak without stuttering for a period of time, although this voluntary fluency may be harder for people with severe stuttering than for those with mild forms of the disorder. In any case, as with the changes in normal speakers, it is difficult for the person who stutters to maintain fluency for a long period of time. In fact, some researchers have reported that as the period of voluntary fluent speech gets longer and longer, there is an increasing need to just let the stuttering come out (B. Guitar, personal communication, March 3, 1993).

What Stuttering Is and Is Not

When people stutter, they do something that listeners can recognize as unusual, even deviant, behavior. It thus is evident that stuttering behaviors differ from normal discontinuities in some way that listeners can perceive. It is not simply that stuttering is extraneous to the speaker's intention, because this is true for normal discontinuities as well. In addition to being simply extraneous to the intention, stuttering behaviors are both excessive and unusual. They are excessive in two ways—they occur more frequently, on the average, than normal discontinuities, and they are, on the average, longer in duration (Bloodstein, 1987; Sheehan, 1974). These two characteristics, plus some others, suggest that what makes stuttering behaviors different from normal discontinuities is the amount of physical and mental effort that they add to the act of producing speech. In addition, some stuttering behaviors are unusual, that is, very different in form from normal discontinuities (Starkweather, 1987). As Van Riper (1982) put it, stuttering calls attention to itself, distracting the listener from the intended message.

Another approach to understanding stuttering is a consideration of what it is not. In this section, we will present some of the common misconceptions about stuttering and show why they are inaccurate.

First, stuttering is not the opposite of fluency. Although fluency varies in both those who stutter and those who do not, it is somewhat misleading to say, as some theorists have, that there is a continuum of fluency, with people who stutter at the low end, say, newscasters at the other, and ordinary "normal" speakers in the middle. Stuttering presents a number of characteristics, among which is the excessive and unusual behaviors described previously. Fluency, which is a characteristic of normal and abnormal speech, can vary from one extreme, in which persons speak exactly what they intend, with no extraneous elements, to the other extreme, in which there are many discontinuities. If stuttering was just a set of behaviors, it would be at the opposite end of this continuum. But stuttering is much more than behavior; it is a cluster of characteristics that includes certain emotional and cognitive reactions. Indeed, it is often said that stuttering is like an iceberg in which the visible part (i.e., the behaviors) are the smallest part of the problem (Sheehan, 1970). In addition to these considerations, it should be noted that stuttering and fluency are not opposites. In professional discourse, the word stuttering refers to a speech disorder, whereas fluency is a skill of speech production that varies in both those who stutter and those who don't.

Second, stuttering is not a disorder of language. Although there is a relationship between stuttering and language (Starkweather, Gottwald, & Halfond, 1990), stuttering is not a primary disorder of any linguistic process. Language use may be influenced by stuttering, and linguistic knowledge may influence the development of stuttering (see below), but the person who stutters seems to be as adept linguistically as the person who does not stutter.[1]

There are some reasonable arguments against this position from people who stress the importance of the role of language in stuttering development (see, e.g., Wall & Myers, 1995), but it remains true that adults who stutter know exactly what they want to say, construct sentences as sophisticated and complex as those of people who do not stutter, and have vocabularies as extensive.

Third, stuttering is not a disorder of voicing, although here, too, there is evidence to the contrary. Many people who stutter block laryngeally, and these blockages often accompany oral stuttering behaviors. The role of voicing in speech production is pervasive, so it often seems that vocal blockages are the nexus of the problem. As stuttering develops, certain vocal reflexes, such as the Valsalva maneuver (Parry, 1994), which causes the glottis to become even more tightly closed as subglottal air pressure increases, may create additional complexities.[2] Also, some individuals who stutter learn to stimulate the airway

---

[1]There is some evidence that children who stutter are slightly delayed in their development of language (Kline & Starkweather, 1979).

[2]The Valsalva maneuver is a semireflexive behavior in which the vocal folds are pressed tightly together in order to hold air in the lungs and build up pressure for lifting, childbirth, etc.

dilation reflex or alter the quality of voicing by letting all their air out as a maneuver to break free of a closed glottis. There are persons who stutter who do not block vocally (Ford & Luper, 1975), and, most compelling of all, there are (although it is a rare phenomenon) individuals who stutter whose larynges have been removed surgically for the treatment of cancer and who go on stuttering afterwards in their esophageal or electronically aided speech (Tuck, 1979; Wingate, 1981). Anecdotal accounts of stuttering-like phenomena in nonspeech mechanisms, as in sign language (Montgomery & Fitch, 1988), playing a musical instrument (Meltzer, 1992), handwriting (Roman, 1959; Scripture, 1909; J. Swaney, personal communication, August 25, 1995), or other manual behaviors (Borden, 1982) also make it clear that stuttering is more than just a voice disorder. Although the voice is vital to speech production and therefore central in many stuttering behaviors, the evidence does not seem to compel the conclusion that stuttering is exclusively a problem of laryngeal control (Starkweather, 1982).

At its most basic level, stuttering is a disorder of speech production. The *primary behaviors* of stuttering manifest themselves at the level of speech motor control (Zimmermann, 1980). This means that when a stuttering behavior occurs, it is the movements of speech that are abnormal, not some more central (e.g., linguistic or cognitive) process nor some more peripheral (e.g., anatomical) variation. It is the movements of people who stutter that are quantitatively different from those of nonstutterers (Klich & May, 1982).

This does not mean that thoughts and feelings may not be a part of the picture or, for that matter, that they cannot influence speech production. They can and do have such influence. Furthermore, these differences in speech motor control can be observed at levels more internal than overt behavior. Specifically, differences between those who stutter and those who do not can be observed in the levels of movement coordination (Caruso, Abbs, & Gracco, 1988; Caruso, Conture, & Coulton, 1988) and muscle activity (van Lieshout, Peters, Starkweather, & Hulstijn, 1993). It must be noted that none of these findings are suggestive of etiology because many different etiologies can result in these disrupted patterns of movement, coordination, and muscle activity.

Many coping behaviors, such as foot-tapping, eye-blinking, or word substitutions, and certain specific emotional, attitudinal, and cognitive differences that typically accompany stuttering are clearly in reaction to stuttering behaviors. Some of these same attitudes and emotional states also clearly exacerbate stuttering. Thus the possibility exists that stuttering can feed on itself in a vicious cycle.

All of these characteristics—additional behaviors, behaviors that last for too long or are too muscularly tense, and the mental and emotional accompaniments of them—point in one direction. They compel the conclusion that what makes stuttering a problem, and what makes it different from the speech of people who do not have the disorder, is that the person who stutters uses too much effort to produce the same syllables that the nonstutterer uses. This does not mean simply that the person who stutters is trying too hard; it means that what listeners react to as abnormal is the extraneous effort that this person uses and the time the extraneous effort occupies.

Severity of Impairment

Stuttering can exist at quite different levels of severity, and this strongly influences the nature of the disorder. When the behaviors of stuttering are infrequent, brief, and unaccompanied by substantial reactive behaviors, thoughts, or feelings, the problem is classified as mild. As behaviors occur more often, are longer in duration, show signs of struggle and tension in the vocal tract, or are accompanied by stronger feelings in reaction to the problem—anxiety, shame, fear, self-hatred, low self-esteem, and so forth—the disorder is considered more severe. It is most important to realize that the primary and reactive aspects of the disorder are independent of each other. Some people with behaviorally mild stuttering have very strong feelings about it; others whose stuttering behaviors occur relatively frequently or are long in duration seem not to be bothered by them very much.

Measuring Severity

Although there is little agreement about how to best measure the severity of stuttering, there is agreement that the frequency with which stuttering behaviors occur is a measurable element of severity (see, however, Young, 1984, for descriptions of the difficulty of performing these measurements). The duration of behaviors also detracts from the time that it takes individuals who stutter to say what they want, and it usually is included in a measure of severity. Similarly, the rate of speech is an aspect of general fluency levels and can play a role in the severity of stuttering. The extensiveness of defensive reactions—both behaviors such as foot-tapping, eye-blinking, facial contortions, and vocal changes and the feelings that motivate and typically accompany them—are an additional element of severity. Finally, the extent to which the person succeeds in avoiding stuttering behaviors detracts strongly from the visible manifestations of the disorder. Unfortunately, no means are currently available for assessing the successfulness of avoidance behavior.

What Is Stuttering and What Causes It?

These are the two questions that people who stutter want answered most often. If we look very closely at what happens when people stutter, it appears that one universal characteristic is an excessive level of muscle tension just before and during the episode, which subsides, but only partially, when the episode is over. Although some attempts to test for high levels of muscle activity in people who stutter have not always been successful (Armson, 1991; Smith, 1995), others (Freeman & Ushijima, 1978; van Lieshout, Starkweather, Hulstijn, & Peters, 1995) have documented well that muscle activity levels are high during stuttering. The location of this extra tension seems to vary from one individual to the next (Ford & Luper, 1975); thus, the structures involved in stuttering behaviors will be different from one person to the next also. This admittedly simple theory of stuttering (Starkweather, 1995b) explains a substantial proportion of the literature, but it does not explain everything that is known about stuttering. Further tests will need to be run before it can be fully accepted.

In any event, the simple theory doesn't explain very much; it just describes what is obvious. To understand a little more deeply what stuttering is, we need to consider the development of the disorder, a task taken up in a later chapter. Nevertheless, we can say here that very young children usually begin repeating whole words and whole syllables with little or no extra muscle tension, become frustrated at their inability to move forward in their speech, and start to try to push in order to force the word out. This pushing is not effective; words come out best when they are not pushed. This counterintuitive concept is hard for preschool children to grasp, so they push. A number of things can then happen. The child can push even harder, provoking his or her speech mechanism into even more muscle tension, with tremors and blocking at the larynx. Other children develop a pattern of avoidance as they learn ways to get around the problem. Some children's parents react to the problem in ways that signal to the child that stuttering is to be avoided. A number of other, even more highly individual, things can happen. One child will develop one pattern of behavior with certain accompanying feelings, whereas a different child will develop another pattern. Many children, perhaps as many as half of those who stutter, somehow find their way out of this problem without professional help, but the rest do not (Ingham, 1984).[3] If the habits of struggle and avoidance and the resulting bad feelings continue on into the time when the child goes to school, the whole complex pattern seems to become locked into his or her automatic production of speech. *Plasticity of development*[4] begins to decline at about this time, and the problem becomes chronic.

Two things are important about this scenario. First, most of the behaviors of stuttering are contained in the reactions of the child to the problem. The whole-word and whole-syllable repetitions without struggle are relatively trivial. It is the reactions that make up most of the disorder. Second, these reactions are accumulated through a development process that is unique to each person. Most of what comprises stuttering is unique to the individual. There are, of course, certain common patterns and tracks. We are all human, sharing characteristically human ways of reacting to things. Under these circumstances it is impossible to say what causes stuttering, and what it actually is, without describing the particular individual's history of development. In other words, there is no single etiology, but as many etiologies as there are stories of stuttering development. Nevertheless, many researchers continue to search for a single cause, an effort that, in our opinion, will never be rewarded with success.

---

[3]Determining what proportion of children who stutter will spontaneously recover is a complex matter. Early studies (Sheehan & Martyn, 1970) were retrospective and, therefore, based on memory. Their findings of very high recovery rates (75% to 80%) based on this flawed methodology were almost certainly too high. More recently Yairi (1992) conducted a longitudinal study showing that the age of the child is of primary importance in determining this percentage. Within 3 months of onset, there is a very high probability of spontaneous recovery. After the child has been stuttering for 3 months, the probability of recovery begins to decline, slowly at first, then faster and faster. By the time a child has been stuttering for a year or more, the chances of spontaneous recovery have declined substantially. Methodological problems in Yairi's study, however, make it difficult to accept the results unquestioningly.

[4]Plasticity of development refers to the tendency in young children to develop in many different ways. As children grow older, this plasticity is lost. In language, the loss of plasticity can be seen most clearly in the acquisition of regional dialect, which can take place in less than a month in a 3-year-old who has gone to another region on vacation, yet eludes adults or even older children who have moved to a new location and would like to sound like natives.

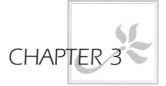
Characteristics of Stuttering and People Who Stutter

People who stutter are a heterogeneous lot. Because stuttering seems not to have a single etiology but is instead the product of each individual's own pattern of development, there is wide variety in the behaviors these people perform, the thoughts and feelings they have, and the ways in which they come to see the communicative world. Although there is less variety within any individual who stutters, the disorder does tend to be complex. Occasionally, a few people who stutter will have simple behavioral profiles, but this typically is not the case.

Stuttering Behaviors

Types

Among the various behaviors that may be demonstrated by people who stutter, the most common and the most characteristic are *repetitions* of speech elements. These repetitions may vary in length. The average duration of a stuttering repetition is 1.6 seconds; however, the standard deviation is 3.0 seconds (Sheehan, 1974), indicating that some repetitions are very long. Repetitions may also vary in the length of the repeated unit. Phrases, words, syllables, smaller parts of words, and simple sounds may be repeated. Typically, the shorter the unit, the longer the person has been stuttering (Bloodstein, 1960). Repetitions may be primary behaviors or they may be secondary. A repeated syllable, as in *"suh, suh, suh,* something," is likely to be a primary behavior, although any struggle that accompanies it may be secondary. A repeated whole word, *"like, like,* like this," may also be either primary or secondary. Many young children have these simple, whole-word

25

repetitions, and in these cases the behavior is probably primary. But adults who stutter often learn to repeat a whole word or phrase so as to stall for time before saying another word, which they are afraid they will not be able to say without stuttering. For example, a person fearing that he or she might stutter on the word "lawn" might say, "Yesterday, I, I, I mowed *the, uh, the, uh, I mowed the, the,* the lawn." The feared word may or may not be stuttered when it is finally produced.

Prolongations are as the name suggests, a lengthening of a sound—either a vowel or consonant—so that its duration is (a) longer than typical, and (b) noticeably deviant from the expected duration of the sound. The average duration of prolongation is 0.87 seconds, with a standard deviation of 0.72 (Sheehan, 1974). The average length is shorter than that of the repetition and, most notably, the standard deviation is small, indicating that, unlike repetitions, the occasional very long prolongation is nearly nonexistent. Only continuant sounds—s, f, th, sh, v, z, w, r, l, y, and all the vowels—can be prolonged.

Blockages are fixations of the airway so that air cannot flow. Although they can happen at any point of articulation (bilabial, labiodental, linguadental, palatal, velar, or glottal) they are far more common at the glottal location, presumably because voicing is a pervasive aspect of speech production. Some authorities (Wingate, 1964) have classified blockages as "silent prolongations," but this is misleading. The term prolongation is most logically reserved for behaviors in which there is airflow and sound. Blockages typically are silent because there is no airflow; thus, they are physiologically distinct from prolongations and should be categorized separately. Researchers who adopted Wingate's erroneous system occasionally reached incorrect conclusions because they categorized blockages as prolongations.

Broken words are relatively brief blockages that occur in the middle of a vowel. After a moment of blockage, the vowel begins again, "li- ike this." The laryngeal tension is quite audible in broken words at the point where the vowel begins again. This reinitiation of the vowel is usually very abrupt, with a nearly click-like quality, indicating the air pressure that has built up behind it.

Tremors are rapid fasiculations of the speech muscles without, or with very little, accompanying movement of the part the muscle serves. Typically found in the person with advanced stuttering, tremors are unlike other stuttering behaviors in one very important way—the person who does not stutter cannot imitate them. They seem even more involuntary than the other behaviors.

Characteristics

All of the behaviors just mentioned can be performed in a wide variety of ways, and certain characteristics describe this variation. One of these characteristics is *tension*. A syllable may be repeated easily or it may be repeated with tension. A prolongation may be easy or it may be tense. A broken word may be released with an explosion of glottal air, or it may be released with a softer impact. This quality seems to be related to the amount of struggle the person feels as he or she tries to get past the stuttering behavior and on with the rest of the sentence. Very likely, this quality of tension arises out of the frustration that people feel as they try to talk, only to find themselves repeating words, sounds, or syllables and unable to go forward and communicate their intention.

A second characteristic is *tempo*. Repetitions may be made rapidly or slowly. There is a tendency for the tempo of repetitions to speed up with development, and it seems reasonable to guess that the speaker speeds the repetitious elements up in order to get past the stuttering behavior and go on with what he or she wanted to say. So the tempo of repetition, like the tension in repetitions, prolongations, and broken words, seems to develop out of early frustration with not being able to express oneself as quickly as one would like.

Coping Strategies

In addition to these behaviors, there is a very large variety of strategies that stutterers adopt to deal with them. These coping strategies may all be considered avoidance behaviors in the sense that they are all motivated by a desire to minimize the stuttering event in some way, although they do not always succeed in avoiding anything.

By definition and by empirical demonstration, frustration is an increase in the force and effort of responding (Amsel & Ward, 1954; Kimble, 1961). Many young children who stutter, frustrated at not being able to move forward and say what they want to say, try to push the word out with additional air pressure. Besides simply pushing, very young children, in their innocent unawareness of what others think, will sometimes jump up and down or hit themselves. Some children will try to pull the words out of their mouths with their fingers or squeeze the side of the cheek to extrude the word. At older ages, children learn to pretend that they don't know the answer to questions, substitute for the upcoming difficult word one that is felt to be easier, or avoid the whole speaking situation if possible. Many school-aged children who stutter hit on a variety of "tricks" that get them out of the stuttering—odd movements of the jaw, eyes, whole head, fingers, or limbs may help for a while.

Any rhythmic behavior will promote fluency temporarily when it is performed so that the production of the syllable can be timed with it. In addition, slower speaking will usually promote fluency, as will more rapid speech if the person uses liberal coarticulation, that is, talking loosely and not very intelligibly. Alterations in vocal quality, pitch, or loudness will also help to avoid stuttering for a time, as will changes in the breathing pattern. In short, almost anything that a person can do to talk differently[1] will, for a while, reduce stuttering. But none of these things, with the possible exceptions of slower rate and word substitution, have been found to be effective in the long term. After talking in a different way for a while, the individual who stutters will find that the stuttering begins to return as soon as the new way of talking begins to become automatic.

A young man whom the senior author met in New York City illustrates this point beautifully. This young man had stuttered since childhood. As a teenager, he discovered that when he spoke with a British accent, which he was quite good at imitating, he did not stutter or at least stuttered much less. A move to a different high school made it possible for him to explain the British accent by devising a whole new life history for himself that included being born and raised in England. Unfortunately, the effect of this avoidance strategy began to wear off as he approached his senior year. He began to stutter once again, even when he spoke in the British accent. Fortunately, however, when he went away to college he was able to entirely reinvent his life history as a person born and raised in France. Of course, with this history went a classic French accent, which reduced his stuttering once again. I lost touch with this young man as a result of moving myself, but I have often wondered what became of him. Did he go on reinventing himself and taking on new accents from all over the world, or did he

---

[1]In order to promote fluency, speech has to be "different" *for the person*. A New Yorker may imitate a Southern accent to be fluent, but the Southerner who stutters might want to adopt a New York accent for the same reason. This is a fascinating phenomenon. It suggests that stutterers will be more fluent when they talk in ways *other than the way their speech developed naturally*. It is further evidence for the idea that stuttering becomes locked into the natural speech patterns as the plasticity of development for speech is lost in the early school years.

eventually realize the futility, or come to hate the dishonesty, of so much effort and deception simply to avoid stuttering?

Categorization Schemes

Many schemes for categorizing stuttering behaviors have been set forth. A very important distinction is one between reactive behaviors and nonreactive behaviors. *Reactive behaviors* are things the person who stutters does in reaction to perceived or anticipated stuttering or its negative consequences. They are defensive reactions:[2] Trying to push the word out, changing the pitch of the voice, slowing down, tapping rhythmically with the feet or hands or nodding the head rhythmically, taking a deep breath, mentally removing one's self from the situation, changing the shape of the face, blinking the eyes, and so forth, are all the things that many people who stutter do in reaction to their stuttering. Some of these reactions are discovered more or less by accident when these people are very young. They discover that these are ways to hide the stuttering behaviors and avoid the shame and embarrassment of stuttering overtly.

Nonreactive Stuttering Behaviors

When the struggle and avoidance behaviors are removed, what is left? To what is the child or adult who stutters reacting? If we look at the earliest behaviors of very young children who later have trouble with stuttering, we often find that they have gone through a period of excessive whole-word and whole-syllable repetition before they began to react (Bloodstein, 1960), although there are some who do not seem to go through this stage but begin to block and stutter in more severe ways right from the beginning. Excessive whole-word repetitions in a 2- to 4-year-old child are not normal. In his study of 2-year-olds who did not stutter, Yairi (1982) found that most of them spoke with less than 4% of their words produced dysfluently, making them only slightly less dysfluent than normal adults. However, excessive

---

[2]Defensive behaviors are defined by Bandura (1969) as behaviors that serve the purpose of preventing the occurrence of or minimizing unpleasant or aversive events.

whole-word repetitions are not exactly abnormal either. Some researchers (Starkweather et al., 1990) chose to describe these behaviors as "at risk" behaviors. Others term them stuttering and still others call them normal nonfluencies for the very young child. In any case, these behaviors do not seem to be reactions to anything. Possibly, they are the 2- to 3-year-old's equivalent of the filled pauses "um" and "uh," sounds that signal the intention to communicate without the readiness for it and tell the listener not to interrupt. Filled pauses do not appear in children until 5 to 6 years of age (Kowal et al., 1975), so it is possible that the very young child repeating whole words is simply recycling through the portion of the utterance that he or she has programmed while waiting for the rest of the utterance to be programmed for production.

The distinction between reactive and nonreactive behaviors is somewhat like another distinction—that between core and secondary behaviors—but they differ in two ways. First, the idea that certain behaviors are "core" behaviors seems not well documented. (See, for example, the intensely critical comments of Adams, 1975, and Freeman, 1975, to Schwartz's 1974 article "The Core of the Stuttering Block.) Second, it is very well documented that much of what people who stutter do when they stutter is react to various stimuli: Stimuli from the environment and stimuli created by the other behaviors that they are performing. Thus, the idea of reaction seems well warranted from the literature, whereas the idea of a core type of behavior does not. An advantage to the reactive/nonreactive distinction is that few assumptions are made about any particular type of behavior. The possibility is left open that some of the behaviors that are often described as core—repetitions, prolongations, and blockages—may themselves be reactive or partly reactive. This fits existing knowledge better than an assumption that, for example, all repetitions are of one kind. There are very clear, substantial differences between repetitions—some are rapid and some are slow, some fragment brief units of speech, others fragment larger units. Some are very tense muscularly, others are not. It seems likely, based on what we know about development, that some of these differences, such as the fragmentation of units, the speed of the repetitions, and the extent of muscular tension, are aspects of repetitions that are attributable to the person's reaction to the behaviors he or she is performing. Consequently, the distinction between reactive and nonreactive behaviors seems more descriptive and less assumptive than the core/secondary distinction.

The reactive/nonreactive distinction is also similar to the distinction between primary and secondary behaviors. But the terms primary and secondary suggest that there is more linearity to the development of these behaviors than seems warranted by observation. A child may initially have whole-word repetitions without struggle and then begin, in frustration, to try to speed up the repetitions and force them out, but the forcing and struggle are part of the repetition. He or she changes the nature of the repetition, but it would still be classified as a repetition. Yet, the forcing and struggling aspect of the repetition seems secondary to the unstruggled repetition, so the primary/secondary distinction becomes muddied in trying to describe such a (very common) situation. Clearly, the forcing and struggling is in reaction to some aspect of the earlier type of repetition, so it seems more descriptive to speak of the one aspect as reactive and the other as nonreactive.

Perhaps the most important point to make is that in reacting to his or her own behaviors, a person who stutters doesn't always add on a new behavior. Often, the reaction simply modifies the character of a behavior that already exists, as in the example of tense and struggled repetitions given previously. Another child may prolong vowel sounds, but as the prolongations take up time and frustrate the child in his or her attempts to speak, he or she may begin to tense the vocal folds, causing the vocal pitch to rise in a siren-like way during the prolongation. The pitch rise is a reactive modification of the prolongation.

Variation in Reactive Behaviors

As mentioned previously, when a 3-year-old child feels that he or she is unable to get words out, a typical reaction is to push harder by compressing the abdominal muscles, as in shouting, but at the same time trying not to say the word louder. The result is complex and somewhat individual. Some children manifest a rising pitch of the voice, others *do* get louder during the dysfluency. A few children block completely, with the vocal folds locking shut. Such a block may last for a few milliseconds (not an insignificant duration) or for several seconds (an eternity in speech terms).

An adult who stutters has reactions that are even more complex, carrying as they do the accumulation of all previous experiences with stuttering. Adult reactions, like those of children, combine the use of force or struggle to get the word out without producing an obvious signal to the listener that such a struggle is going on. The adult's reaction thus also contains two forces that are incompatible—a force to push the word out, to go on, to say the word and then the sentence that follows it, but at the same time not to reveal to listeners any sign that there is a problem. This simultaneous pushing out and holding back was identified years ago by Sheehan (1970) as a form of approach-avoidance behavior.

Characteristics of the Person Who Stutters

Stuttering is more than just repetitions, prolongations, and pauses. It is the inner and outer struggle to be fluent. As David Shields' book *Dead Languages* (1986) so clearly exemplifies, the struggle to communicate is at the heart of the human condition, and, in this way, stuttering mirrors something that is intensely and uniquely human. Van Riper (1982) also touched on this theme when he described stuttering as the "dark mirror of communication." Benson Bobrick, in *Knotted Tongues* (1995), described it this way:

> Stuttering is an affliction that renders defective the uniquely human capacity for speech. In its severest form, it can be a crippling disability; and of all disabilities, it is perhaps the least understood. The dignity of the person, his distinctive humanity, and even his soul, as made manifest in rational discourse, was (and is) by tradition, associated with speech. Together with the capacity for thought that it expresses through language, speech defines us as human more adequately than any other faculty we have. Its deprivation—in stuttering, its audible and visible disintegration—cannot but be felt as a catastrophe. (p. 23)

We are all struggling to express ourselves. Perhaps that is why the people who do not stutter seem to react with fear and anxiety in the presence of stuttering (Wingate, 1971). They know the fear of not communicating from their own dysfluencies (White & Collins, 1984) and in this way are no different from the person who stutters. Just a tilt of the genetic Pachinko game, a microscopic DNA aberration, might put the listener in the place of the person who stutters.

Some individuals try to hide their stuttering from the world. At the one extreme are people for whom the discovery of their stuttering by listeners is the worst possible thing that could happen. They order food they do not want in a restaurant because they know they will stutter on certain sounds. These are people who will exchange the word they want to say for another, easier word. They say "Yes?" when answering the telephone instead of "Hello." Many have adopted nicknames designed to avoid a dreaded sound in their actual name. They pay a high price for not letting their stuttering show. Those who change words can become so involved in the process of finding the easier word to say that their language becomes vague and convoluted. They sacrifice clarity of expression or their preferred food, and with it some self-esteem, to avoid exposing the stutter.

An extreme example of this was a young rabbinical student who worked with the senior author. This young man spent much of his time reading, but he often had incorrect prescription glasses because, during the ophthalmological examination, he would say the letters he could *say* instead of the letters he could *see*. As a result, his glasses were seldom correct.

Other people have found hiding to be futile and allow their struggle to be visible. They may have decided that there is little point in trying to hide the stuttering and, as a result, their struggle is overt. They push and force and struggle until the difficult word is produced. They tap their feet, blink their eyes, nod their heads, or slap their legs. These behaviors are forms of defensive reaction.

Emotional and Cognitive Reactions

The emotional and cognitive reactions to stuttering are important to recognize. Emotional reactions range from petty annoyance to stark humiliation and shame. In between are varying degrees of frustration, anxiety, anger, embarrassment, and fear. Cognitive reactions to stuttering include faulty attributions ("I am a poor speaker"), rationalizations ("If only I didn't stutter, then I could . . ."), minimizing ("It isn't that bad"), and unfounded perceptions ("They are all laughing at me").

We list these reactions here not to demean the character of people who stutter, but to emphasize that these are among the many ways of defending one's self against the psychological pain of the disorder. It is often these and other forms of denial that needlessly prevent the person who stutters from being fully aware of his or her behaviors, thoughts, and feelings. The result is a perpetuation of the problem.

A remarkable form of avoidance/denial common in people with severe stuttering and in other survivors of early trauma has no formal name but could be called "losing touch." The person who stutters in the middle of a block experiences a diminished awareness of his or her surroundings. Some researchers say that these individuals feel as though they are blacking out, yet they know they will not lose consciousness. They lose awareness of where they are, what they are doing, to whom they are talking, or any of the details in their immediate environment. They have left the moment. Some see themselves from afar. A young woman for whom English is a second language described on STUTT-L her "out of body experience" this way:

> Normally I don't think that much and don't feel that much while stuttering because I'm often "out of my body" by that time—so to speak. I don't quite know how to explain this, it's a defense of mine; when there is something difficult I'm in the air, I don't feel anything and can't think. My energy isn't in my body but flying above my body, [it seems]. It's just the very opposite of being grounded. I think I do this while stuttering because at that time I don't have to feel what I feel (shame, I think, for instance) and to realize what I think. I think there is anger in me, anger out of frustration. I sometimes realized in the past that I was angry with myself when I stuttered and was calling myself names, which I did do often but I decided to stop that.
>
> [Recently] I've become more aware of "being out of my body." Also I've become aware that when I'm kind of aware that I'm not that much in my body when I stutter I *refuse* to come back. I just don't want to feel what I feel and think what I think.
>
> "Flying" is so exciting and it feels like my whole life is more exciting. The negative aspect of "flying" is fear and panic for all kinda things and situations—and fear for life itself I daresay. I'm struggling with this issue the last few weeks. After a long period of more or less "flying" I now am more in my body and more on the ground (yes and find life rather boring). (A. Stelwagen, personal communication, October 2, 1993)

It is clear from her description that "flying" is a defense against the pain of experiencing her stuttering completely. It is, after all, the mind that is in pain at these moments, and the mind has the amazing capacity to just go and be somewhere else, a little farther away, where it doesn't hurt so much. It should hardly be surprising that many people who stutter find themselves using this device.

A number of personality traits, found also in individuals who do not stutter, may play an important role in stuttering. Amster (1995) surveyed people who stutter at a meeting of the National Stuttering Project and via the Internet. Matched controls were also surveyed. Overall, although the sampling in this study was not random, and as a result the conclusions have to be qualified, Amster found that the people who stutter scored higher on the perfectionism scale than people who did not stutter, both when they assessed themselves currently and when they looked retrospectively at their level of perfectionism in earlier years. Figure 3.1 shows Amster's results. This does not mean

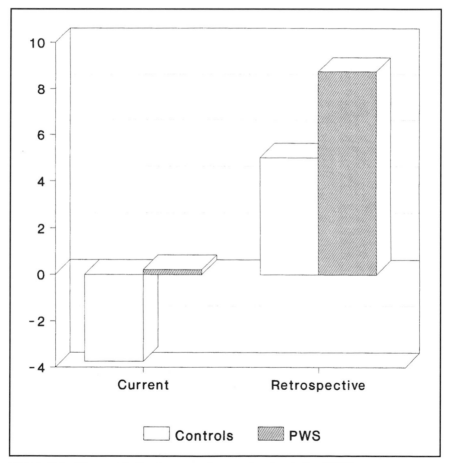

Figure 3.1. Mean perfectionism score for people who stutter (PWS) versus non-stuttering controls. From "Perfectionism and Stuttering," by B. Amster, 1995, in C. W. Starkweather and H. F. M. Peters (Eds.), *Proceedings of the First World Congress on Fluency Disorders: 1994*, pp. 540–543, Nijmegen, The Netherlands: University of Nijmegen Press.

that all people who stutter are perfectionistic, only that for these individuals the average tendency toward perfectionism is greater than for people who do not stutter. Amster defined perfectionism as not accepting failings in performance or character. Her preliminary conclusion was that those who are perfectionistic from the beginning are more likely to try to hide, avoid, or do battle with this disorder than those who are less perfectionistic. In this way, the trait of perfectionism increases the likelihood of reactive behaviors.

Related to perfectionism is the strong need many people who stutter have to control their speech. They try very hard to "make it right." This kind of control stems from fear. When the struggle to control an errant tongue, jaw, glottis, or diaphragm is exacerbated by the fear that what will come out if it is not controlled will embarrass, shame, or humiliate the speaker, there is a natural surge of muscle tension that seems to make even more likely the tremors, blockages, repetitions, and prolongations that define the disorder at a behavioral level. Again, a personality trait—in this case the need to control—may serve to abet the development of the disorder in some people. Of course, whatever the type of personality, it will have an effect on the way an individual stutters and the types of avoidances or defense mechanisms that are used. In short, every aspect of the disorder can potentially be influenced by the personality.

Exacerbating Features

Time pressure is naturally a major problem for many people who stutter. Stuttering behaviors occupy time without conveying additional information, and, as a result, the speaker is not keeping up to the norm for information flow in a conversation. He or she begins to say a sentence with the idea that the sentence will take a certain amount of time, but then, perhaps with no warning at all, a word takes two or three times longer to get out than he or she would have thought, so time has flown away and the pressure to make up for it begins to mount. Given a number of stuttering behaviors within an utterance (and stuttering behaviors do tend to cluster together, one behavior begetting another as it were), this time pressure mounts up quickly. Any external source of time pressure only makes this worse, so standing at a counter in a fast-food restaurant while there is a line waiting puts even more time pressure on the speaker. Answering the telephone, when there are only a few seconds to say "hello" before the caller says "Hello? hello? Is anyone there?" is also a time-pressure situation. Saying one's own name is the highest time pressure of all. Hesitating, even for a second, makes it look as though you don't know your own name. This particular type of situation thus tends to be quite difficult for most people who stutter. Another time-pressure situation is the block that lasts too long. As soon as a block or a stuttering behavior has lasted beyond a certain point, the speaker senses that he or she is just taking up the listener's time unnecessarily and may decide then to force the word out with some bizarre or extreme behavior.

Related to time pressure is a sense of urgency that many people who stutter have. It may be that dealing with all this time pressure leaves these individuals with a sense of "speech urgency," a need to communicate that is stronger than that found in other people. As a result, they may tend to interrupt more often than they should or talk much more than they should. Perhaps this is also a product of the frustration they carry with them of never being able to say what they want. When they finally get the floor, they may hesitate to give it up. In this and other ways, people who stutter often lack some of the knowledge of pragmatics[3] that other people take for granted. Growing up with a communication problem as severe as stuttering can be, often shortchanges a person in the experiences from which a knowledge of pragmatics develops.

Recursion and Paradox

One of the most intriguing and puzzling things about stuttering is its *recursion*. Hofstadter (1979, p. 128) has described recursion as "nesting, and variations on nesting . . . [stories inside stories, movies inside movies, paintings inside paintings, Russian dolls inside Russian dolls (even parenthetical comments inside parenthetical comments!)—these are just a few of the charms of recursion.]" One of the most well-known examples of recursion is the statement "This sentence is false." Is it true that the sentence is false? Or is it false, and therefore true? The

---

[3]Pragmatics refers to the aspect of language use that is concerned with the choice of language forms (words, terms of address, structures) that vary according to the social situation.

problem is that the sentence refers to itself and modifies itself and in so doing operates on itself. Another common example is the internal loop in a computer program. When a loop is introduced, the program is said to "push" down to a new level. A series of nested loops is called a stack. The words "stack," "push," and "pop" come from the way dishes in a cafeteria are stored in a spring-loaded device that "pops" up when a dish is removed and "pushes" down when a dish is placed on top of the stack. The metaphor is helpful in understanding the nature of nested loops. As Hofstadter (1979) put it,

> To push means to suspend operations on the task you're currently working on, without forgetting where you are—and to take up a new task. The new task is usually said to be "on a lower level" than the earlier task. To pop is the reverse—it means to close operations on one level and to resume operations exactly where you left off, one level higher. (p. 128)

Stuttering is a recursive system, operating on itself and modifying itself; as a result, it can often create a stack of behaviors, thoughts, and feelings inside other behaviors, thoughts, and feelings. For example, on the behavioral level, a young child may say, "Mommy, *can, can, can, can,* can I go to the bathroom?" The series of repeated words is a kind of loop through which the child's speech production mechanism cycles for reasons we do not know. A high frequency of these loops during sentence production can frustrate the child's natural desire to communicate. As a result of the frustration, the child may try to force his or her way through the words, triggering a Valsalva reflex and causing the vocal folds to clamp shut in a blockage. "Mommy, c[block]an I go to the bathroom?" At this point, the blocking loop is nested inside the word-repetition loop, but because time passes during the block, and the reason (maybe word finding, or uncertainty) has passed, the system also pops out of the word-blocking loop and into the repetition loop when the block ends. It then pops again out of the word-repetition loop, at which point the sentence is completed.

Another child, trying in frustration to escape the word-repetition loop, might fragment the repeated words and produce "Mommy, *cuh, cuh, cuh, cuh, cuh,* can I go to the bathroom?" In this case, the system pushes down to a word-fragmentation loop, which cycles until the moment has passed, then pops back up to the rest of the sentence. But both the blockage and the part-word repetition are themselves just as frustrating as the original whole-word repetition, so in anticipation of the repetition, the child might push down to an even lower level in which a stall for time or backing-up loop is entered, as in "Mommy, *uh, mommy, c-, uh, c-, uh Mommy* . . . " then pops up to finish the sentence. But of course the backing up also takes up time, and the child may push down to even a further level by avoiding speech—"Mommy . . . "—then rushing out of the room in the direction of the bathroom. There is more. The child may now figure out some way to avoid the whole process—not asking permission, for example—and at the same time seek to avoid all the really unpleasant feelings of embarrassment, humiliation, and fear that he or she knows will accompany attempts to ask. Figure 3.2 illustrates the nested loops and levels of recursion.

Nested loops like these in a person's speech-production system create a very tight knot that the person who stutters may find very difficult to untie. When the system is pushed down into a third or fourth level, it is hard to know just where you are or what to do to get back to actual speech production.

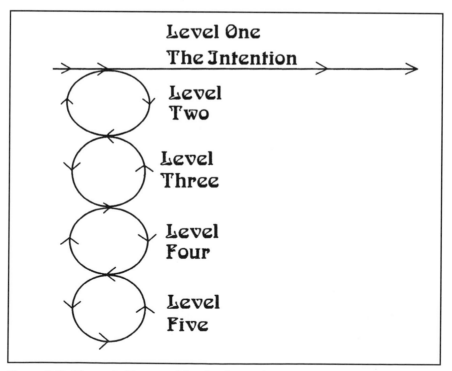

Figure 3.2. The nested loops and levels of recursion.

Often, when there is recursion, paradox is not far behind. As in the statement "This sentence is false," paradox is when two things are simultaneously opposite; the sentence is both true and false at the same time. In stuttering, paradox has a more concrete expression. The person is trying to talk but, at the same time, is trying not to stutter or is trying to make up for the time lost to stuttering. Stuttering is a way of talking, however, and both stuttering and talking take up time. Thus, the person who stutters is simultaneously trying to talk and trying not to talk, trying to make up time but losing time in the process. Sheehan (1970) advanced a similar position when he described stuttering as an approach–avoidance conflict. Whether it is approach–avoidance or the paradox that results from trying to talk recursively, it is no wonder that the person finds him- or herself entangled in an underbrush of words, behaviors, thoughts, and feelings, unable even to see a pathway out into a clear meadow of easy talking.

Additional Sources of Variability

As previously discussed, stuttering is an unusually variable disorder at the behavioral level. Some individuals who stutter repeat initial sounds or whole words; others prolong initial sounds; still others break words with an abrupt cessation of voice in the middle of a vowel. Others block silently with the vocal folds, the lips, or the tongue, temporarily frozen to the point of articulation. In some people, the stuttering behaviors are very long in duration, whereas in others they are brief. In addition, the behavioral defensive reactions—foot, hand, or finger tapping; head nodding; gasping for air; suddenly exhaling; jerking open the jaw; jerking the head backward; using facial grimaces, hand or foot movements, or writhing of the torso; changing the quality, loudness, or pitch of the voice; substituting words that are easier to say fluently for the difficult words, stalling for time to let the tension pass—vary even more widely from person to person.

This very wide variability in behavior means that clinicians and laypeople alike often encounter stuttering that doesn't sound the way they think stuttering should sound. For example, one person who stuttered never repeated and prolonged sounds or blocked, but, as he anticipated that stuttering was about to occur, he could change the quality of his voice to a more breathy, hoarse sound and continue to talk this way until he was past the difficult sound. He sounded like someone with an intermittent hoarse voice, but he was a person who stuttered.

Perhaps even more extreme are the people with "covert" stuttering: People who have become so adept at word substitutions that they never stutter overtly at all. It is not uncommon for such an individual to carry the secret of his or her stuttering alone, with no one among friends or family aware that an inner struggle to speak in a normal-sounding way is always present. This person is an extreme example of avoidance, illustrating, as only an extreme example can, something about the nature of the disorder. Sheehan (1970) described stuttering as an iceberg, with most of the disorder hidden from view. In the person with covert stuttering, *all* of the disorder is hidden from view. This suggests that the important aspects of the disorder are the parts that are unobservable, as Sheehan noted. Sheehan argued vociferously, if not bitterly, against the radical behaviorism that prevailed in the 1970s. He would be gratified to see that today it is his view that has prevailed.

Fluency-Enhancement Conditions

Stuttering also varies in that in many, but not all, cases, it is alleviated, or even removed entirely under certain specific, externally imposed conditions. When these conditions are removed, stuttering returns. These "fluency-enhancing conditions" are similar in certain ways, but different in others, and it has been a major research effort to discover what they might have in common. Such a discovery would be important in determining what kinds of things influence stuttering.

The main fluency-enhancing conditions include the following:

talking very slowly
talking in chorus with another person
talking with delayed auditory feedback (DAF)
talking with frequency-altered feedback (FAF)
talking under loud background noise
talking while whispering or initiating speech in a whispery voice
talking in time to a metronome or other rhythmic stimulus
talking to a nonjudgmental listener
talking with the voice at a different pitch
talking in a dialect not one's own
talking while playing a role
saying material with little content or importance
saying familiar material

These conditions are listed roughly in the order of their effectiveness, with the most effective ones at the top of the list. Some conditions of speech combine several of these conditions. For example, singing combines slower rate, pitch alterations, familiar material, and perhaps a changed role.

The reasons for these fluency-enhancement effects are not entirely clear. Wingate (1976) reviewed most of them and came to the conclusion that what these effects had in common was a change in vocal functioning. However, for some of these conditions, he had to stretch quite far to find the change in vocal functioning. For example, during choral speaking such a change can occur, but it doesn't have to, and later research (Adams & Ramig, 1980; Kalinowski, Armson, & Stuart, 1995) showed that the fluency-enhancing effects of choral speech could occur even without vocal changes. Similarly, Garber and Martin (1977) demonstrated that the fluency-enhancing effects of masking noise were independent of changes in vocal functioning.

Van Riper (1963) believed that these effects were attributable to a distraction from the morbid attention to dysfluency itself, but this "distraction hypothesis" was later disproved by research showing that, at least in the case of talking in time to a metronome, an irregular rhythm, which ought to have been more distracting than a regular one, actually had less of an effect on fluency than the regular rhythm (Fransella & Beech, 1965).

Other authors (Starkweather et al., 1990; van Lieshout et al., 1993) speculated that it was a change in motor patterns that was responsible, but this idea also seemed uncertain because some of the fluency-enhancing effects, such as FAF, appeared not to alter the speech patterns, at least not in any obvious way. Andrews et al. (1983) examined the most powerful of the fluency-enhancing effects and concluded, although somewhat tentatively, that a combination of slowed rate and externally supported timing control produced the effect. However, a recent study by Kalinowski et al. (1995) showed that fluency enhancement via FAF could occur "in the absence of slowed rate," and, in addition, the frequency-altered feedback effect seemed to function by giving the person who stuttered the illusion that he or she was speaking in chorus with another speaker[4]; in fact, he or she was generating

---

[4]Interestingly, the devices that are available on the market that amplify the voice of the person who stutters probably function in the same way, even though some very elaborate theoretical notions have been suggested to explain them. People who use these devices say that it makes them feel as though they are talking in chorus with another person.

the choral signal. This challenged the idea that the fluency-enhancing effect of choral speech depends on the external support of the other speaker. In FAF, the "other" voice is that of the person who stutters. At this time, a generally accepted, completely explanatory position has not been taken.

These altered ways of talking, either with or without external support, have formed the basis of a number of treatments and devices (see "Devices that Reduce Stuttering" in Chapter 7), but there is virtually no evidence that the effects of these treatments are anything but transitory. Some of the treatments based on these effects do not claim that the fluency-enhancement effect is going to be long-lasting. Instead, they put the individual who stutters under the fluency-enhancing condition and then slowly wean him or her from that condition to the more variable and unpredictable conditions of everyday speaking. Unfortunately, the stuttering usually returns in a while.

In addition to these specific situations, most people who stutter are more fluent when they are less anxious. In young children, it is not just anxiety, but also excitement, that tends to make them stutter more. This raises an interesting point. If children stutter more when they are very excited, which is a positive emotional state, *and* when they are anxious, which is a negative emotional state, what can be concluded about the effects of emotion on stuttering? Clearly it is not simply that people stutter when they are anxious. A reasonable conclusion is that it is the heightened state of muscular tonus in the speech mechanism that these two emotional conditions provide (Starkweather, 1995b).

Parents of children who stutter and adults who stutter are often quite puzzled by these effects. It often reinforces the erroneous notion that stuttering must be a "psychological" problem. For the adult who stutters this can quickly turn into doubts about one's own mental health. One individual we know had an unusual, but not unique, pattern to his stuttering. When he blocked severely, he could feel his anal sphincter tightening in synchrony with his vocal mechanism. This is not a particularly unusual reaction, because the Valsalva maneuver reflexively co-contracts anal and vocal muscles. But, in the psychoanalytic tenor of the times, it made the person think that he had a deeply disturbed psyche in which vocal and anal functions were somehow connected. He didn't really feel as though he were deeply disturbed; in fact, he felt pretty normal psychologically, as he was, but every time he blocked on a sound he was presented with evidence to the contrary. It took many years of introspection and a great deal of money spent on psychological testing and therapy before this person learned about the reflexive connections of the vocal folds and the anal sphincter and was absolved of these serious doubts about his mental health.

Speech clinicians who are familiar with the literature on stuttering and understand the true nature of some of these phenomena can help people who stutter understand that they are no more insane or neurotic than the rest of the population.

Another interesting effect is that of the nonjudgmental listener. Most adults who stutter will say that their speech is much improved when they talk to a listener who is nonjudgmental and open about stuttering (Laris, 1994). A very common example of this is the fact that most people who stutter are at their most fluent when they are talking to a speech clinician. The ease with which they can talk to a listener who is open and nonjudgmental about stuttering behaviors is actually part of a larger picture: The tendency of stuttering to be diminished under conditions in which stuttering is desirable. The latter of these effects, the open and nonjudgmental listener or, in a general sense, any condition in which stuttering is accepted, can produce dramatic effects (see the section on Paradox earlier in this chapter).

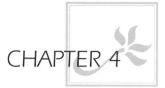
Course of Development

S tuttering usually begins slowly, and almost imperceptibly at first, typically in quite young children. The results of seven studies on stuttering onset (Andrews & Harris, 1964; Berry, 1938; Darley, 1955; Johnson, 1955; Johnson & Associates, 1959; Milisen & Johnson, 1936; Preus, 1981) are shown in Figure 4.1. The youngest, oldest, and average age of onset are shown for each study. It is clear that, on the average, stuttering begins between the ages of 4 and 6 years. It is also clear that stuttering can begin in older children, as the oldest age of onset in the seven studies ranged from 11½ to 15 years. However, this later age of onset is considerably more unusual than a younger age. The youngest ages of onset in each of the studies was less than 2 years. Furthermore, because the average is closer to the youngest ages than to the oldest ages of onset, it can be seen that a greater number of children were in the group whose stuttering began at ages younger than average than in the group with an older than average age of onset.

Early onset of stuttering is therefore not only possible, but somewhat more likely than later onset. Furthermore, it is not true, as has often been thought, that the very youngest children who stutter are "going through a phase." Yairi's (1992) data show clearly that children who do not stutter are only slightly less continuous in their speech production than adults, and any clinician who has seen a reasonable number of people who stutter can report that very severe symptoms can occur in very young children. The youngest child ever treated by the first author of this book was 15 months old, toddling around in diapers, repeating words and syllables, pushing and forcing out words, giving up on speech attempts, and even jumping up and down to get his words out.

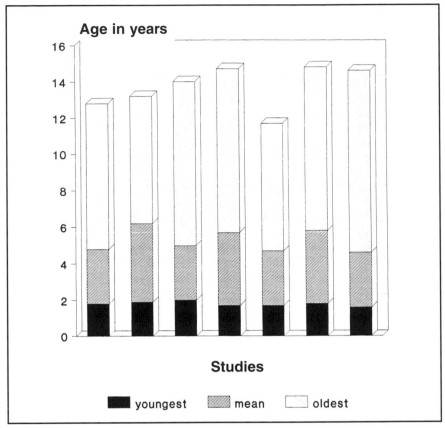

Figure 4.1. Seven studies of onset.

General Trends in Stuttering Development

Stuttering is a disorder that involves changes in distribution over time and space. Although both the pace and the course of development are highly individual, there are some predictable patterns (Bloodstein, 1960). In addition, the development of stuttering is superimposed on the development of the person (Peters & Starkweather, 1990a), which is true for adults as well as children because humans are always growing. When stuttering develops in a child, it is not just the child that is developing and changing, but also the child's family. When stuttering comes along, it alters the child; however, the family reacts to it, and this alters certain aspects of the family and family life. These changes in turn may be something to which the child reacts, so that the stuttering behavior changes, often becoming worse, which makes the family react again. It is clear that as stuttering develops in children, two other developmental systems are intimately involved—the child as a person and the child's family (Meyers-Fosnot, 1992).

Increased Severity

Two general trends of development can be identified. The first pattern is a tendency for stuttering to become more severe over time. This retrograde development is most evident in the early years. In spite of this general tendency, there are typically periods of stability—times when nothing is changing—which become longer as the person becomes older. There are also children in whom stuttering does not become more severe but stops spontaneously.

The tendency for stuttering to become more severe over time in the earlier years of its development seems to result from the child's reaction to the problem. Each reaction makes the problem worse, which in turn increases the reaction. It is in this way that new behaviors, conglomerations of behaviors, and increasing tension in existing behaviors add to the growing severity of the problem. This is not to say that every child reacts badly to the presence of dysfluency in his or her speech. Some children probably find dysfluency to be no more than a petty annoyance, but those who are not troubled by the presence of dysfluency probably do not become people who stutter, so it is difficult to obtain information about these children. Others may react initially to dysfluency in a way that makes the problem worse, but through their own intelligence and wisdom, or through the intervention of their parents or someone else, they come to realize that their initial reaction was not helping and take a new direction, which is eventually successful in routing them away from the problem. It is only those children whose reactions are maladaptive (i.e., that tend to make the problem worse) who go on to have chronic stuttering. In some cases, it appears that there is a process that makes the maladaptive reaction itself more likely to recur.

Changes in Distribution of Behaviors

Temporal Distribution

The second trend involves changes in the distribution of stuttering behaviors over time and space. In the very young child, stuttering (or at-risk behavior) comes and goes. Episodes of stuttering may last for several days or several weeks, then seem to disappear (Bloodstein, 1960). This can be confusing for the parents, who often alternate between outright panic during an episode to relief and a false sense of complacency when the episode is over. A typical scenario is for a parent to call a speech clinician and, in a state of considerable distress, request an evaluation. The appointment is made, but by the time it comes around the problem has completely disappeared, and the appointment is cancelled. In some cases, when the appointment is not cancelled, the child is brought in but no stuttering behaviors can be observed. Under these latter circumstances, many clinicians make the very serious mistake of telling the parents that there is no problem, or, if there is, they can't see it and therefore there is nothing that can be done about it. The wise clinician explains the episodic nature of early stuttering to the parents and counsels them on the assumption that there really is a problem, at least one of risk.

These episodes of stuttering/fluency gradually smooth out into a somewhat more stable pattern in which stuttering is present but rises and falls in severity. In 30% to 50% of the cases, the at-risk behavior stabilizes into normal speech behavior (Ingham, 1984). But in the rest the possibility for a lasting episode of normal speech becomes less and less likely as the child gets older.

Spatial Distribution

There is also a change in the distribution of stuttering with regard to space. In early stuttering, the disorder tends to occur with approximately equal severity in all situations. In the adult, however, it tends to occur in some situations with more severity than in others, and there are often situations in which the person doesn't stutter at all. This is called *situational dependency* or *situational specificity*. The transition from the young child who stutters with roughly equal severity in all situations to the adult with a clear pattern of situational dependency usually begins within the first few years after onset.[1] Once developed, the situation in which the child is talking begins to influence how much, or even if, he or she will stutter in that situation. The behaviors seem to become "attached" to particular listeners, particular

---

[1]An exception to this is the child whose stuttering begins suddenly and with substantial severity. In these cases, it will be attached to the same situation almost from the beginning.

words, words that begin with particular sounds, or specific speech situations, such as talking on the telephone, ordering in a restaurant, asking questions, saying one's name, or talking to strangers or authority figures (see Starkweather, 1996, for a discussion of this process).

Both the smoothing out of episodes and the attachment of stuttering to specific situations are related to development, and both seem to reflect the influence of learning in the development of the disorder. The tendency for the disorder to come and go wanes as the problem becomes more and more an internalized difficulty, something that is part of the child's speech pattern and thus more pervasive. Situations become stuttering-eliciting stimuli because of the association that they develop with the experience of stuttering. So, the experience a child has struggling to talk to his or her father makes it more likely that the next time he or she talks to the father something similar will happen. It is not necessarily related to the father's behavior; however, if the father reacts negatively (e.g., punishing the child for stuttering or repeatedly telling the child to slow down or take a deep breath) future stuttering will be elicited in his presence.

Development Through the Life Span

As people grow their capacities change, and the environment changes, too. These environmental expectations come not just from listeners, but from the person as well. Children come to expect certain things from themselves, just as adults do.

H.F.M. Peters and Starkweather (1990a) examined the development of stuttering throughout life, and identified five phases of development, as follows:

Phase 1	2–6 years	Preschool Period
Phase 2	6–12 years	Early School Years
Phase 3	12–17 years	Puberty and Early Adolescence
Phase 4	18–30 years	Later Adolescence and Early Adulthood
Phase 5	30+ years	Maturity

These phases occur in both the development of stuttering and in the development of capacities and demands for fluency. It is probably no coincidence that the development of stuttering closely parallels the development of motoric, linguistic, socioemotional, and cognitive capacities.

Phase 1

The first phase is characterized by very rapid development in all areas. The child with normal speech typically has acquired sufficient linguistic skills by age 2 years to make essential wants known and to comment on the surrounding world. As the child progresses through this period, a developmental "explosion" occurs in all areas of language—syntax, semantics, pragmatics, and phonology. As a result, by the end of the preschool period, the child is speaking in sentences that are (a) syntactically close to those of an adult, (b) semantically adequate for the child's immediate purposes, and (c) phonologically intelligible. The drive for language development is essentially unstoppable.

Supporting this explosion of linguistic growth is a more moderately paced development of speech motor control that in general manages to keep pace, at least in the typical child, with language development. As sentences get longer, however, they are also spoken more quickly and require a more complex motor plan for execution. Children at this age frequently stumble in their speech as their motor system races to catch up to the burgeoning number of words and sentence forms. For some children the motoric job is too difficult, and an unusual amount of dysfluency occurs, which is noticeable by those who know the child and frequently is a cause for concern.

Social, emotional, and cognitive skills are also improving during this period. Children develop a confident anticipation of the future, including confidence in their ability to express themselves, and an awareness of the consequences of all of their actions, including speech. During this phase, most children overcome the shyness that keeps them clinging to their parents. Crying is less frequent as well.

In the area of cognition, children learn that speech is something that they do with their mouths, throat, and lungs. In the early years of this phase children know little about speech, complaining that "the words have little hooks on them." In addition, when words do get stuck, Phase 1 children are quick to use a strategy that works to solve many of the other problems that children of this age encounter—they push harder. If something is stuck (e.g., a toy wedged into the corner of a playpen or a tricycle in a pothole), pushing and forcing are a typical preschool child's type of solution. They do not yet have the capability to consider solutions that involve gentleness and slow movement (e.g., petting a cat). They grab, hold on, and stroke, a little too hard, until the cat manages to get away. So it is with speech. If the word is stuck in a child's mouth, he or she pushes it out; if it doesn't come out right away, he or she pushes harder. Such a strategy may trigger vocal tract reflexes, such as the Valsalva maneuver, that lock the vocal folds even tighter, so that sound cannot be produced. Similarly, pushing and forcing may also make the oral muscles tense to the point where they cannot move in the smoothly coordinated way that speech production requires.

Phase 2

In Phase 2, the child begins school, and language skills become more refined, particularly in the area of pragmatics and phonology. Vocabulary also continues to increase, as it will throughout life. In the early school years, however, language development is much less impressive than in the preschool years.

Motorically, an important change occurs in the late preschool or early school years. The child begins to automatize speech motor control, as evidenced by the achievement of speech that is nearly as rapid as that of an adult and consistently smoother than it was in the preschool years. The advantage to this automaticization of speech is the new freedom the child has to think about the ideas that are the content of his or her communication. Surely one of the wonders of the evolution of speech is this ability to have the vocal tract do all that complicated work with little or no thought; yet, the use of speech and language for communication could not have evolved in any other way.

There is a price paid for this remarkable motor skill. As speech production becomes more and more automated, it also becomes less and less capable of change (Krashen, 1973). The loss of plasticity of development that accompanies the development of semiautomatic speech motor control is a small price to pay in most cases, but when the speech patterns reach this stage and still contain erroneous phonological or fluency patterns, the increased difficulty in correcting these disorders can become a very heavy price to pay.

The school-age child's social, emotional, and cognitive abilities are characterized primarily by a changeover from the influence of parents and siblings to that of peers. This extraordinary social and emotional occurrence makes the early-school-age child difficult to influence and/or change, unless the change requested happens to coincide with the perceived approval of the child's school friends. During this phase, the increased importance of peers and the substantially larger amount of time the child spends with them create opportunities for comparison. The child now sees him- or herself not just as separate from his or her parents, but as a part of a social group, and it becomes important to the child to be considered to be like the others in the group. As a result, a sense of strengths and weaknesses, and of competition with peers, begins just as the approval of peers becomes important. For the child with a stuttering problem, this means that there is the possibility of teasing. Teasing occurs in younger children, too, but it lacks importance. The younger preschool child draws his or her strength from parents, and the occasional jibe from a playmate doesn't matter if there is acceptance at home. Now that the child is in school, the acceptance or rejection of the peer group is much more important, and teasing becomes a major social crisis for the child who deviates from the norm. It is at this age that a profound loss of self-esteem can occur for the child who is different from his or her peers. Tolerance of differences among classmates will not develop until Phase 3.

Because of the growing importance of peers during this phase, the child who stutters is likely to develop an attitude that anything is better than stuttering. If there is any behavior than can be performed that will prevent the stuttering behavior from occurring, or that will extricate the child from the humiliating moment, it will be acquired, held onto, and used. The discovery of one of these "tricks" is a moment of great delight for young school children. They believe they have found the solution to a problem that has been frustrating their attempts at communication for a number of years.

The child's deviant behavior, and the many unusual things that he or she has to do to cope with it, can create a deep sense of difference and shame. When this shame is amplified by parental shaming as a behavioral control tactic, or when the parents themselves feel ashamed of the child when talking to a third party, the child's sense of self-doubt and self-hatred can reach profound depths.

Phase 3

In Phase 3, motoric and linguistic developments are slow, and the skills that support fluency are relatively stable. The one exception to this is the pubertal changes that occur in vocalization, particularly in boys. It is of some theoretical importance that these dramatic changes in the functioning of such a pervasive aspect of communicative behavior as voicing hardly ever have an effect, for good or ill, on the young person who stutters. If stuttering were primarily a problem of vocalization and phonation, we would expect to see a dramatic surge in the number of onsets of the disorder as this important structure becomes temporarily unstable. Instead few cases of stuttering that begin during adolescence have been reported, and young people who stutter already usually manage pubertal voice change with no effect at all on their stuttering behavior.

Socially, however, there are profound changes during adolescence that mostly revolve around the person's sense of identity. In addition, there is a growing realization that soon he or she will have to take a place in the adult world. As a result of these changes, and because of the increased sexual awareness that makes necessary the use of speech and language in a new way—the dating scene—a problem such as stuttering suddenly becomes more serious. The person realizes that it can pose a real threat to vocational and romantic success. Later, he or she will discover that romance, dating, marriage, and family are not much threatened by stuttering, but during the adolescent years, a young person who stutters too often gives up on the possibility of ever having a normal social and romantic life.

When it comes to obtaining work, however, they can be quite right. Stuttering often poses a huge barrier to acquiring a job. Discrimination in the workplace in hiring, promotion, and retention is very widespread (see Chapter 1). These realizations change the way the person views his or her problem, and they can often lead to serious attempts to overcome it, with or without speech therapy.

Phase 4

In Phase 4, the stability of motoric and linguistic skills continues, but the social and emotional changes that began in adolescence continue on into young adulthood. The person's sense of identity becomes much more firmly established and, for those who are still stuttering at this time, the tendency to identify themselves as people who stutter is now more fully developed. There is also an increased emphasis on family life and the acquisition of more advanced knowledge and specialization in the workplace. Many people who stutter learn that they can do whatever it is they have chosen to do in spite of their stuttering problem, but many others will avoid careers where they think speech will be important.

Phase 5

In Phase 5, general motor skills are beginning to decline, but speech motor skills remain intact and can continue at a very high level until very late in life. At the age of 92, the actor Sir John Gielgud read a lengthy passage of Oscar Wilde's on the occasion of that writer's belated interment in the Poet's Corner of Westminster Abbey. Gielgud's voice and interpretation were scarcely less powerful than they were at the height of his career when he was in his 50s. Of course, we are not all John Gielguds, and some decline, most particularly in speech rate and in phonation, may occur. In general, however, speech motor skills remain competent until late in life.

This motoric stability is accompanied, finally, by a corresponding emotional and social stability. Perhaps because of this stability in all of the areas affecting stuttering, there is a tendency in many (but not all) people who stutter at this phase for the disorder to become less severe. The tricks and avoidance behaviors often are abandoned during this phase (or earlier) as "excess baggage," and productive attempts at recovery are often made. Later on, there may be a crisis of self-confidence and regrets over paths taken or not taken earlier, but even this midlife crisis seems not to have too much effect on stuttering.

It can be seen, then, that as a person develops through the life span, his or her skills, perceptions, and beliefs also change, and these changes affect the nature, and sometimes the severity, of the stuttering problem. It also appears that an unfortunate sequence in which slowly developing speech motor skills may bring on the disorder, only to be followed by unsettling periods in the development of emotional maturity, prevents the solution of the disorder through most of childhood. Speech clinicians who evaluate children and adults who stutter will benefit by fitting into the picture of symptomatology a sense of the person's life history and life stage.

Tracks of Development

Van Riper (1973) identified four distinct tracks, or commonly recurring patterns, of development: (a) The garden variety, in which nothing unusual was happening in the child's life, and onset was gradual at a young age (2½ to 4 years); (b) later onset accompanying poor articulation; (c) later onset following a traumatic incident; and (d) later onset with awareness but no avoidance. In the first author's clinical experience, there are six discernible tracks of development.

Track 1

The first track is *garden-variety stuttering*, which is by far the most common. In this track, as in Van Riper's Track 1, nothing unusual is happening in the child's environment; the stuttering seems to develop without warning and with no environmental events—stress or excitement—that could account for it, but the child's development of speech and language is otherwise normal. There may or may not have been a family history of stuttering. The parents may well react to the child's dysfluency with fear or some other negative emotion, but often they seem to react with the kind of care and support that any speech clinician would want. There is no clear explanation of what has happened except that the child has started to stutter. Typically, the stuttering begins with easy whole-word repetitions and progresses slowly to struggle and forcing.

Track 2

The second track, which is the next most commonly occurring one, is found in the child whose communicative environment is characterized by a high level of verbalization. His or her parents talk all the time, value talking highly, and may place a negative evaluation on silence. These *language overstimulation* cases (Amster, 1989), mentioned previously in the discussion of linguistic demands on fluency, occur often in the children of people who are in professions characterized by a high level and a high quantity of verbal activity (e.g., lawyers, speech pathologists, salesmen, preachers, or teachers). The children are usually younger at the time of onset, sometimes extremely young. Many are under 2 years of age. They are predominantly characterized by having language development that is advanced for their age, often extraordinarily so, and in our experience somewhat more than half of them have been girls. Their parents may be extremely delighted in the precocious development of their language, or, in some cases, they may have sought to directly correct the child's use of language at a younger age than is typical. (Direct correction is more typical of a 7- to 8-year-old child's parents.) The children struggle very hard to talk correctly from the beginning. There is no period of easy whole-word repetitions, as in the garden-variety type of development. Their speech motor skills and their general motor skills are normal for their age.

Track 3

The third most commonly occurring track is demonstrated by the child whose language development is *delayed* and who is placed in *language-stimulation therapy.* As a result of the therapy, this child's language develops rapidly, and he or she often reaches normal levels of language development. However, just as these children begin to seem to have recovered from their delayed language development, they begin to stutter. Usually the stuttering occurs on linguistic forms, or on words associated with linguistic forms, on which they have been working. Both the language therapist and the parents are typically delighted at the progress in language development and are correspondingly horrified at the appearance of stuttering. Struggling is present from the beginning. These children tend to be a little older and are more likely to be boys than girls.

Track 4

The fourth track is very much like the third, except that the problem is *articulation.* The child is slowed in phonological development and is placed in therapy for it. This therapy usually is partially successful, although the great success seen in the language-delay cases does not occur in these cases. When stuttering appears, it is often in concert with the exact same sounds on which the child has been working. It thus seems to be the same as Van Riper's Track 2. If is common in children with Down syndrome, who often have poor articulation and try hard in speech therapy to learn how to produce the sounds of speech more intelligibly. The problem is that they try too hard; the additional muscular effort they use to produce the sounds they find difficult seems to directly result in stuttering on those same sounds.

Track 5

The fifth track is similar to Van Riper's Track 3, in that it is characterized by a *traumatic experience* or a *prolonged period of stress.* From the beginning, this stuttering seems brought on by stress or change. Most young people who stutter respond not just to anxiety, but also to high levels of excitement, and this is also true for this group of children. Many young people are particularly sensitive to changes such as a new school or a move to a new location, but the experience doesn't have to be a negative one. In one case, a little girl began to stutter when she first saw her parents after an extended absence. The "trauma" in this case seems to have been the sudden rush of happiness and relief at seeing them home again. It should be noted that there is no period of easy whole-word repetitions in this group.

Track 6

In the sixth track is found the child who seems *delayed in his or her ability to control the movements of the vocal tract.* These children are unusually slow talkers for their age; frequently, one of their parents is also a very slow talker. Although they do not struggle very much at the beginning, they begin to struggle soon after onset. These children seem frustrated by the time that stuttering takes up and are most dysfluent in time-pressure situations.

No attempt should be made to read too much into these tracks; they are simply the result of one clinician's observations over a number of years. It cannot be stressed too much that the development of stuttering is determined by the complex interplay of demands and capacities, co-occurring with the child's and the family's development, making it a highly individual matter. Only the initial few behaviors of stuttering look similar across individuals. Each person reacts differently to these behaviors, however. As he or she continues to struggle with the problem, with the family also getting involved, the problem becomes increasingly more individualized. When one considers that the early behavior is the tiniest fraction of the problem, and that 98% of what makes stuttering a problem for a speaker is in the experience-shaped reactions to that problem, and the layers upon layers of reactions that occur afterward, it is no wonder that the disorder is different in each person who has it. It is not just that there are multiple causes: There are as many causes as there are people who stutter because the real cause is the pattern of reactions that the person brings to it. The apparent tracks probably result from the fact that many children share similar experiences; parents often react to stuttering in similar ways; and certain types of experiences—language therapy, articulation therapy, trauma, and advanced language development—have a tendency to promote dysfluency in children.

Genetics and Stuttering

Finally, it is quite evident that stuttering runs in families. The evidence is rather compelling for a genetic, rather than a strictly experiential, explanation (Kidd, 1980), although experience plays a highly important role in the development of the disorder. It is not known, however, what inherited trait leads one child to develop chronic stuttering while another child does not. It could be that children who inherit superior language skills (except for those who have been overstimulated at a young age) have the tools with which to recover from stuttering. Or it could be that some children inherit poor levels of speech motor control that predispose them to stuttering. It is also not known if the genetic influence is present in all individuals who stutter. There are people who stutter who have no family history of stuttering.

Twin studies shed some light on this situation. Howie (1981) discovered that identical twins were concordant[2] 90% of the time, whereas fraternal twins were concordant only 25% of the time. This suggests that genetic factors play a role, but not the only one, in determining who will develop stuttering. It should be remembered, however, that a developing child tends to create an environment around him or her, and identical twins are likely to create a similar environment; thus, the experiential versus genetic question is not perfectly answered by the study of twins. Nevertheless, the difference between 90% and 25% is large and compelling, and this, in combination with the results of other studies (see Kidd, 1980), makes it very clear that genetic factors

---

[2]Concordant means that both twins share the trait in question, in this case, stuttering.

play an important role in the development of stuttering. For example, in twins who have been separated and reared apart, there is a very low concordance. Farber (1981) found that in five pairs of twins reared apart in whom at least one stuttered, *none* were concordant. Although this is a small number of participants on which to base conclusions, and the data were taken from reports of twins separated at birth, rather than from a more scientific sampling technique, they neverthe-less suggest that experience plays a powerful role.

The evidence quite clearly indicates that both genetic factors and experience play a role in the development of stuttering. On reflection, this should not be surprising. In most human behaviors, genetic fac-tors determine the constraints and capacities of a physiological sys-tem, the perceptual abilities, and, to a certain extent, the likes and dis-likes. Experience shapes the final behavioral product within these genetically determined boundaries. It seems unlikely that stuttering would be any different from any other behavior in this regard.

Whatever the genetic component of stuttering development turns out to be, and future research may well provide an answer to this issue, it is clear that when one or both parents of a child who stutters are or have been individuals who themselves stuttered, their experi-ence influences their behavior with the child in an important way. These parents often are more sensitive to the problem of stuttering than parents who have not experienced it. They bring their child to the speech clinician within a few weeks of onset, and sometimes are very worried about the child's future. They may also model struggle and avoidance behaviors that the child may acquire through vicarious con-ditioning. However, these parents are also sensitive to what the child is feeling and usually know better than the nonstuttering parent how to support the child by being open and accepting about the problem. They are the clinician's best ally.

Stuttering in the Preschool Child: The Demands and Capacities Model

The Demands and Capacities model (Starkweather, 1987; Stark-weather et al., 1990) dichotomizes what is known about influences on stuttering into two categories: *demands*—those environmental events (including the internal environment) that make the child's fluency diminish—and *capacities*—those qualities of the individual, inherent or acquired, that make the child develop more fluent speech. Each category is further divided into four areas of behavior—motoric, linguistic, socioemotional, and cognitive.

Demands on Fluency

Motoric Demands

Motoric demands include certain environmental[3] events that make it more difficult to move speech structures smoothly and quickly. Probably the most important of these is time pressure. Nearly every person who stutters finds it more difficult to speak fluently when the circumstances require more rapid speech. But some of these circumstances are easy for people who do not stutter to miss:

> Saying "Hello" when picking up the phone
>
> Saying his or her name
>
> Repeating what was just said in response to "What?"
>
> Saying a longer sentence or a longer word
>
> Speaking when everyone is in a hurry, as when it is time to leave for school
>
> Speaking when people are waiting for a response

Some of these situations are also filled with time pressure for the child who stutters, depending on the child's age, but others are unique to the child. Probably the most common one is parents or other significant people in the child's life who speak very quickly. Children try to conform to their families, and when a child is in a family where one or more person speaks very quickly, the child will probably try to talk quickly, too. Sometimes it seems as though one parent is a very slow speaker and the other one is very fast. The child has the slow speaker's genetic endowment, which is not helpful when it is the fast-speaking parent who is present. Not just rapid speech, but rapid turn taking,

---

[3]The word "environment" is used here to refer to the communicative environment, that is, stimuli derived from the communicative setting, including the listeners and the speaker; the physical surroundings; the type of sentence being uttered and the purpose to which it is being put; and the specific word, syllable, or sound being produced, which can have an impact on the speaker's fluency.

which can include actual interruptions, also puts time pressure on a child. In addition, in a large family where there is competition for speaking time with siblings, it is the fast talker who can grab a few seconds of the family's attention. This too is a time-pressure situation for the child.

Linguistic Demands

The various aspects of *language use* that can be demanding of fluency include word finding, sentence formulation, complex phonological combinations, and difficulty in using the appropriate form for the social circumstances. These are the semantic, syntactic, phonological, and pragmatic aspects of language use. When a child is slower in finding words or formulating sentences, the time lost stresses the child's fluency. Phonologically complex combinations can stress a child's immature coordination, and pragmatic demands may raise anxiety levels. In addition to these linguistic demands, language stimulation can stress fluency levels through "language overstimulation" (See the section on Development Tracks earlier in this chapter) or through language therapy.

During therapy for delayed language, it sometimes happens that a child develops stuttering. These cases of stuttering seem to be a result of the therapy, not the original language problem (Merits-Patterson & Reed, 1981) and are described below.

Various aspects of *language knowledge* that can also be demanding of fluency are vocabulary, syntactic knowledge, phonology, and pragmatics. A child with a larger vocabulary may need more time to find or choose words, and a child who knows many complex forms may need more time to formulate them. The time lost can stress the child's fluency. Phonologically complex combinations can stress a child's immature coordination, and pragmatic demands may raise anxiety levels. It may be more difficult to find a word from a larger than from a smaller lexicon, and it may be more difficult to formulate a more complex sentence. Certainly, a higher level of linguistic knowledge presents motoric demands, because the more complex sentences are usually longer and spoken more quickly.

Socioemotional Demands

Two emotional states that frequently make stuttering worse in children are excitement and anxiety (Adams, 1990). These two states have in common a heightening of general muscle activity levels, which perhaps is the reason that they seem to have a similar effect on fluency level, in spite of the fact that they are opposite in valence. Clinicians have noted also that the events that excite or frighten children are not exactly the same as those that excite or frighten adults. Prolonged periods of tension also seem to make stuttering worse (T. Peters & Guitar, 1991).

Cognitive Demands

When a person talks, he or she is moving, thinking, feeling, and constructing language simultaneously, so all four areas of capacities/demands are in use. There is evidence that a demand placed on the motor area can detract from the function of the linguistic and cognitive areas (Kinsbourne & Hicks, 1978), and it has been argued that demands on any area can detract from the function of any other area (Levelt, 1989; H. F. M. Peters & Starkweather, 1990b; Starkweather, 1991). Consequently, when a child is asked to perform a speech act that is accompanied by a more complex thought, the possibility that this may detract from the child's motor performance has to be considered.

Also, children whose cognitive development has reached the point where they can conceive of their speech as a process have a better tool with which to deal with dysfluent speech than children who are still unable to separate their speech from their thought. Thus, the metalinguistic level of development is also a category of demand/capacity.

Capacities for Fluency

To meet the demands of the environment, the child can employ motoric, linguistic, socioemotional, and cognitive skills to achieve fluent speech. Consequently, the four areas covered in the preceding section on environmental demands—movement, language, emotion, and cognition—are the same areas in which children may vary in their capacity for fluent speech. Although the information on demands came from studies in which an environmental variable was shown to affect fluency,[4] the information on capacities for the most part came from studies that showed people who stuttered to be inferior to those

---

[4]In a few cases, such as cognition, very little empirical data are available.

who did not stutter with regard to the skill in question. There is, in our opinion, a somewhat larger inferential leap in the latter case than in the former. Of course, it is necessary to make this leap because we cannot ethically damage or limit children's capacities in order to assess the effects of such limitations on their fluency.[5] Nevertheless, the conclusion that individuals who stutter lack a specific capacity is less well founded than the conclusion that a specific environmental variable is demanding of fluency.

In both areas, there is an additional limitation. Most of the information we have with regard to demands as well as capacities is derived from studies done with adults. This raises the possibility of a specific kind of contamination: The findings of these studies might have been influenced by the person's experience as one who stutters. In the case of capacities, this means that the subject may have been less able to react quickly, move quickly, formulate sentences, and so forth, because of the continued presence of the disability during his or her lifetime. In the case of demands, the adult who stuttered might have developed a certain sensitivity to environmental variables as a result of his or her experience with stuttering. In both cases, the issue is separating cause from effect, always a problem. It is, however, a much more serious challenge to the validity of the conclusions in the case of capacities, where the results already were not certain because the capacity was inferred from the observed difference, in addition to being extrapolated from adults to children, whereas in the case of demands, only the extrapolation, not the additional inference, was made.

Motor Capacities

Motor capacities for speech are the abilities to: (a) react quickly to external stimuli; (b) move the vocal tract rapidly; (c) coordinate the various vocal tract movements with each other, specifically with regard to timing; and (d) move smoothly, that is, to contract muscles without fasciculation.

The ability to react quickly to external stimuli clearly distinguishes individuals who stutter, both children and adults, from those who do not, as the voluminous and robust reaction-time literature shows

---

[5]A recent longitudinal study of children at risk for stuttering (Kloth, Janssen, Kraaimaat, & Brutten, 1995) was not subject to this limitation. This study is described later.

(Andrews et al., 1983). It therefore seems logical to suggest the possibility that rapid reaction is a capacity for fluency. Several problems in addition to those mentioned above make this suggestion somewhat difficult to accept. First, there is no indication that reaction time plays a role in speech production. There are no correlations of vocal reaction time with any measures of speech production—such as speech or articulatory rate, the duration of speech sounds, or other aspects of speech timing—or any of the physiological measures, such as muscle activity level, even though these variables have been shown to be related to stuttering in one way or another. Furthermore, muscle activity, a variable that *is* related to speech production (Armson, 1981) and is clearly elevated in many stuttering behaviors (Ford & Luper, 1975; Freeman & Ushijima, 1978), even during observably fluent speech (van Lieshout et al., 1993), would be likely to slow reaction time. It is possible at least that the slower reaction times of people who stutter are a direct consequence of raised muscle activity in the speech mechanism during its use, an effect of the disorder rather than a capacity for fluency.

It should be noted, however, that reaction time *does* play a role in one very specific aspect of speech production—the speed with which a conversational partner can respond in turn. Although a limited aspect of speech production, getting started is a very common source of difficulty for people who stutter. In this limited sense, reaction time may be a capacity for fluency.

The ability to move the vocal tract quickly has also been identified as a capacity for fluency based on a limited number of studies showing that people who stutter do not move their vocal tracts with the same speed as their peers who do not stutter (H. F. M. Peters, Hulstijn, & Starkweather, 1989; Starkweather & Myers, 1979). Of course, there is no question that the ability to move the vocal tract rapidly can and does contribute to a speaker's articulatory rate. Nevertheless, it is still not clear whether velocity of movement is related to stuttering as cause or effect. Given a vocal tract musculature stiffened by a higher level of muscle activity, particularly when that activity occurs in antagonistic muscles, a slower velocity of movement is to be expected.

The ability to coordinate the various vocal tract movements with each other has been shown to distinguish individuals who stutter from those who do not, but *coordination* has many meanings. Freeman and Ushijima's (1978) observations of simultaneously co-contracted antagonistic muscles could be termed *discoordination*. So too could Caruso, Abbs, and Gracco's (1988) observations of differences in the timing of different parts of the vocal tract during production of a given token. It is probably most helpful to think in terms of entrainment.[6] Entrainment can either help or hinder performance. The pianist who has learned to control his or her finger movements so that they will play music in spite of the natural tendency of the fingers to entrain pinky with pinky and index with index has a developed a high level of coordination. So, too, has the tennis player who has learned to step forward with the left foot while swinging the racket with the right hand, making use of the body's reflexive entrainment of right hand and left foot. The term coordination could also refer to a person's ability to anticipate events in time, perhaps with the aid of some temporal structure such as a rhythm or an arhythmic template, so that movements can be made at the right time relative to other movements. Finally, the consistency of many motoric performance variables— acceleration, velocity, deceleration, duration of steady state positions, relative timing of different structures—and the adjustment of muscle activity during varied conditions in the vocal tract—such as speaking louder or faster—could also be termed coordination. One of the most robust findings in the literature has been the variability in the performance of individuals who stutter as compared to those who do not. In other motor acts, variability can be recognized as a lack of coordination.

In some of the ways just described, people who stutter have been shown to be less coordinated than those who do not. But here, too, it is not easy to distinguish cause from effect, nor is it logically defensible to apply results obtained with adults to the speech of children.

The recent study by Kloth et al. (1995) was extremely well designed and executed; consequently, it is not subject to most of the limitations mentioned previously. These researchers identified as at risk for stuttering a pool of nearly 100 normally speaking children between the ages of 23 months and 58 months for whom one or both parents stuttered. The authors made a number of measures of these at-risk children, including language skills and speech–motor skills. A year later, 26 of the children could be identified as stuttering. The authors then compared the data taken previously on those children who had begun to stutter with those who were not stuttering at that time. They found that the children who would begin to stutter later on talked

---

[6]*Entrainment* refers to the tendency for a movement made with one body part to be accompanied by simultaneous movement of another body part, as, for example, when a person talking moves his or her head simultaneously with the production of stressed syllables.

more rapidly than the children who did not develop any stuttering. However, neither group of children talked at a faster than normal rate. Because both groups in the study were considered to be at risk for stuttering due to a positive genetic history, the authors concluded that the slow rate of children who did not end up stuttering protected them from developing the disorder.

Linguistic Capacities

Linguistics capacities for fluency include the rapid finding of words and the rapid formulation of grammatical sentences. They also include the ability to feel comfortable in saying the right thing on a particular social occasion. These are aspects of language use, or performance, not aspects of linguistic knowledge or competence. Linguistic knowledge—knowing that a sentence is correct or that a word is suitable—is different and was discussed previously in the section Linguistic Demands. (For further details, see the discussion in Chapter 5 on the evaluation of demands and capacities.)

Socioemotional Capacities

Socioemotional capacities for fluency include a person's ability to continue to move slowly and smoothly when excited, anxious, or angry. Because stuttering behaviors often are accompanied by fear, embarrassment, shame, frustration, or anger, the ability to continue talking at the same level of fluency in the face of emotions that tend to charge the speech musculature with tension and tremor is an evident capacity for fluency. (For further details, see the discussion on the evaluation of children in Chapter 5.)

Cognitive Capacities

Cognitive capacities for fluency include the ability to think about speech in a way that separates it as a process from the person performing it. Helpful in overcoming stuttering, this metalinguistic skill is usually present in children shortly after they begin school and in nearly all children by the age of 8 years. Unfortunately, stuttering is typically well established by that time and the presence of metalinguistic knowledge, although helpful, is not sufficient to overcome the disorder. Another cognitive skill is the ability to understand that some things happen better when one doesn't try so hard. At 3 or 4 years of age, when stuttering typically begins, the child lacks the ability to understand this concept. Later, when the child can imagine—or has some experience with—such circumstances, it is too late. The stuttering is already well established.

The Development of Demands and Capacities

As children grow, their motoric, linguistic, socioemotional, and cognitive capacities for generating a smooth and rapid string of syllables naturally increases with continued development. At the same time, however, the communicative environment—their listeners and also themselves—come to expect more mature behavior. As a result, the demands and capacities are increasing at the same time, but not necessarily at the same rate. As long as the child's capacities for producing fluent speech are ahead of the demands for fluency that the child's environment presents, the child will speak fluently; however, when the demands become too great or the capacities have not developed fast enough, he or she will not be able to speak fluently. Because demands vary according to a number of factors, such as the speech situation, the listener, and even certain words and sentences, the child's ability to speak fluently will also vary. As the capacities for fluent speech improve with maturity, the child may well reach a point where dysfluent speech is no longer a problem because all speaking circumstances present demands that are within the child's ability.

Stuttering in the School-Age Child: Learning to Avoid

Shame and Teasing

By the time they reach school age, most children who stutter have a well-developed habit of tensing and forcing as they initiate the process of speech production. Consequently, their speech is noticeably abnormal. In spite of this abnormality, and the fact that the child is struggling to talk, stuttering typically does not present a social problem during the first 1 or 2 years of school (ages 5 and 6). Children have progressed in their cognitive development enough to know that they are individuals, but they have not progressed very far in knowing what kind of individuals they are; because of this limited awareness, teasing is not a major problem in the earliest school years.

By the time they are in school, many children who stutter also have acquired a substantial load of shame. This sense of shame develops out of the reactions, nonverbal and otherwise, of their parents or other significant adults. Parents who wince, roll their eyes, or look disgusted when their child stutters during the preschool years are sending a message, consciously or not, that stuttering is shameful. Parents who are ashamed of their child's stuttering provide an unfortunate model for the child. As the child grows older, he or she often develops a cloak of denial to counter the chill wind of shame.

When these children are still only 7 or 8 and becoming aware that they have strengths and weaknesses as people, the teasing that they get from their peers can be devastating because it reinforces the already present sense of shame. It becomes important at this age to do anything except stutter in front of people. Out of this social desperation, two things develop: One is the sense that they are just not good at talking, and the second is a sense that they are simply not very good as people.

Speech is so closely tied to one's self-identity that to be a "poor" speaker feels very much like being an incompetent person. Of course, these children are no less competent than their peers. They may be good at playing basketball or chess, may have musical talent, or be whizzes at math. Unfortunately, the low self-esteem related to their speech can override all these positive talents. Interestingly, these children are not poor speakers. Their speech lacks fluency—it doesn't come out easily—but their language skills are as normal as the next child's. Their voices are as melodic and clear as that of their peers (unless tension associated with stuttering has made them chronically hoarse). They articulate the sounds of speech as clearly as their peers and pronounce their language with the same facility. They communicate with energy or enthusiasm and express themselves with clarity and élan. It is only that, on some occasions, their speech is peppered with extraneous behaviors and postures and with tension in their vocal tracts. The problem is often considerably smaller than it appears, both to the child and to the parents. A speech clinician can often help to restore the missing perspective by explaining to both parent and child everything that is normal or superior in the child's speech.

Acquisition and Adoption of Secondary Behaviors

The second thing that develops out of the schoolchild's social desperation is a "bag of tricks" to deal with stuttering. It is during this stage that children learn to stall for time, hide, avoid, or escape from the stuttering behavior and its associated shame and humiliation. For example, when a child first discovers that he or she can successfully prevent a repetition or prolongation from occurring by looking up at the ceiling and pretending to be thinking of a word, it must be a wonderful moment. They have only to feign a little momentary ignorance and the stuttering can be forestalled. The same feeling of accomplishment probably accompanies the first time these children discover that they can get their vocal folds to open up by letting out all the air and triggering the airway dilation reflex, or they can change to a word that is easier to say, or they can change their vocal quality to a breathier sound, and so forth. Additional examples include pulling the lips back around the teeth, tapping rhythmically on a nearby surface, bouncing the head rhythmically, jerking open the jaw at the same time as attempting the difficult word, or looking away from the listener to lower the growing sense of fear that they are going to stutter.

In some cases the tricks remain effective. Word changing, for example, seems to continue to be an effective way to avoid stuttering, even in adults. Many of these tricks, however, just lose their effectiveness. Why this happens is a little mysterious. Possibly it is *because* these additional extraneous behaviors become so abnormal that they lose their ability to diminish the abnormality of the original behavior. Research on the natural history of defensive behaviors is sadly lacking.

Often, as the tricks begin to lose their effectiveness, the child will try the same trick in a larger form. For example, a child who has been told to take a deep breath before he or she speaks will find that this breath gives him or her a little time during which the muscle tensions in the vocal tract subside a little, and he or she is then able to talk without stuttering. Then there is a time when the child uses the trick and stutters anyway. To cope with the weakening effectiveness of this trick, he or she enlarges it by taking a deeper breath. This may work for a while. When the deeper breath doesn't work, the child takes an even deeper one, because making the breath deeper restored its effectiveness in the past. The child continues to breathe deeper and deeper, perhaps elevating the shoulders, throwing back the head, and lowering the jaw. The originally innocuous behavior has been shaped by differential reinforcement into a bizarre, almost grotesque addition to the things the child does to get words out.

In this way the secondary behaviors become a part of the extraneous behavior, that is, stuttering, making the problem worse. Because the extraordinary reinforcement they provided in the beginning and the differential reinforcement that shaped them into increased abnormality, they are heavily locked into the child's repertoire of stuttering behaviors. In other words, the disorder creates the disorder. They start out as a way of solving the problem and end up being a part of the problem. Usually, these tricks become a much bigger part of the problem than the original stuttering they were designed to avoid. When the child has become an adult, he or she may come to realize how fruitless all this struggle was; for the time being, however, the child does not want to give up these crutches. There is still hope, which occasionally is reinforced by a positive result, that they will get the words out. During this time, when the child is laboring under misconceptions about what speech is, what stuttering is, and what he or she can do about it, it is difficult to remediate stuttering. The child's own defenses create resistance to treatment, which the wise clinician must learn how to handle.

The Importance of Listeners

The reactions of parents and other significant members of the listening environment that were so important to the preschool child are internalized in the school-age child. It seems to the struggling child who stutters that it is the listener who is controlling his or her speech. These children must come to recognize that when the listener's reactions are more important to them than their own internal values, they have given their power away to the listener. Such a situation allows for the development in these children of fear of, or anger and resentment toward, listeners, as if they created the problem. Listeners do feed into the problem by reacting with anxiety toward and judgment of the person who stutters, but the latter often accepts the judgment as true, believing that he or she is inferior in speaking ability or worthy of critical judgment because he or she cannot do what is so easy for everyone else. Physically handicapped individuals, such as those who are paraplegics, were in the same place 30 years ago, buying into the idea that they were "handicapped." Now they have come to realize that they can do almost anything in the way of work, although they may need some reasonable accommodation and access. In the next few years, it is to be hoped that people who stutter will go through this same transformation.

The Grief Cycle

The development of stuttering in adults can also be described with reference to the grief cycle. In grieving over the loss of a person, a limb, or a function, it is common first to deny the problem and be angry about it, then to bargain, grieve or feel sad, and finally accept it. All of these stages can be present at the same time. The school-age child who is fighting with the stuttering as if it were an enemy is in an anger phase. When people of any age who stutter avoid the problem, they are attempting to bargain with it or deny it. As school-age children reach adolescence, they can begin to see themselves in relation to the rest of the world in a more realistic way. Ideally, they fantasize less and instead accept themselves for who they are, with all their strengths and weaknesses, and begin to think purposefully about how they can support themselves, form long-term relationships, raise families, and so forth. Often, during this time, the denial that motivated the avoidance tricks in the school years begins to dissolve, and the young adult begins to see the problem differently and begins to believe that he or she can do something about it. Bargaining and anger may still be present in one way or another (e.g., the young adult is often interested in quick cures), but it is lessened by cognitive and emotional development.

These changes promote increased self-awareness. The difficult school-age years are over, and the prognosis for recovery is better. Clinicians can capitalize on these tendencies to promote awareness and acceptance of one's stuttering, and, through these steps, open the door to change.

It is through these natural stages of the grief cycle that many adults who stutter find their way into the recovery process, often without any help from speech clinicians. The speech clinician who is judgmental, sees his or her role as one of providing critical evaluation, or attempts to change the person's behavior without first preparing the way through awareness and acceptance runs the risk of alienating the client not just from him or her, but from the whole profession of speech pathology. There are literally thousands of stories of such alienation. It isn't necessary for alienation of this kind to continue. Using the inherent principles of awareness, acceptance, and change, client and clinician can work together, respecting and listening to each other, simultaneously influencing each other, and simultaneously growing. These three stages of recovery from stuttering are discussed further in Chapter 7.

Adult Onset of Stuttering

Two rather rare forms of stuttering develop in adults: psychogenic stuttering and neurogenic stuttering. Because these two types seem to develop almost exclusively in adults, whereas the most common type of developmental stuttering begins in childhood, it can be argued that the two "adult" forms are something quite different—not really stuttering at all, but something that closely resembles it. Questions of this sort are not easily resolved because they depend heavily on the definition of the disorder that one adopts. So in this text, where stuttering has been defined as excessive struggle and effort in the production of speech, psychogenic and neurogenic stuttering both would be considered stuttering, even though one of their chief characteristics is that they do not engender as much effort as does developmental stuttering. Still, because they are characterized by more than a normal amount of effort in the production of speech, they will be considered as forms of stuttering rather than as a separate disorder.

Psychogenic Stuttering

Psychogenic stuttering is caused by an identifiable psychological event. There seem to be two types of psychogenic stuttering: One is associated with a traumatic event or a period of prolonged, intense stress. An example of this posttraumatic-stress type of psychogenic stuttering can be found in the following case history. A 35-year-old man was driving alone on a heavily traveled highway when his compact car was sideswiped by a trailer truck. The truck swerved just before the contact and was teetering on two wheels as it dragged the little car along for 20 to 30 seconds before it came to a halt. The driver of the compact thought that the truck was about to fall on him as he was being dragged along; as a result he was terrified for a prolonged period. Eventually, the two tangled vehicles came to a stop without further incident, and miraculously no one was hurt. The man found his way home about an hour later, where he greeted his wife, and she immediately noticed that he was not speaking normally, but instead was repeating sounds and syllables. She took him to the hospital, where he was given an intense and thorough set of examinations for neurological damage, but none was found. He was uninjured, but he was stuttering. The stuttering persisted after the event for a number of years, but it never changed in form. The man continued to repeat whole words and the first syllables of words about 15% of the time without any sign of struggle, forcing, or avoidance. He was annoyed by the stuttering, and frustrated by his inability to communicate easily, but he was not ashamed, embarrassed, afraid, or angry about it. He simply accepted it as a consequence of his accident.

The other type of psychogenic stuttering is associated with a conversion reaction, which is a specific pattern of reaction to an emotional conflict in which the resolution of the conflict is avoided by the occurrence of some physical symptom. Often the word hysterical is used to describe conversion reactions, although this use of the word does not conform to contemporary everyday usage. Other forms of conversion reactions are better known because they are more common than stuttering. For example, in World War II, a number of cases of *hysterical aphonia* (loss of voice) were reported in officers who found themselves in a battle situation in which they would have to give orders that would cause men to die. The sudden loss of the voice avoided the necessity of giving the orders. Hysterical deafness also occurs as a conversion reaction when a person is faced with the necessity of hearing something extremely unpleasant or terrifying. Hysterical stuttering is quite rare: Only a few cases have been reported. In one, a young woman was in a very bad marriage, and she knew that in order to end the situation she would have to confront her husband and explain to him why she intended to leave him. The conflict went on unresolved for a considerable period of time. She just could not bring herself to say the words. Eventually, she started to stutter. Somehow, at least in her mind, the stuttering relieved her of the responsibility of having to say the awful words to her husband (Roth, Aronson, & Davis, 1989).

Neurogenic Stuttering

Neurogenic stuttering is a symptom—usually one of several, that follows injury to the brain. The injury may be from a blow to the head, a stroke, or the result of a disease that attacks the neural tissue. Stuttering is more commonly the symptom when the injury is more diffuse rather than associated with a particular area of the brain. This type of injury is more common following brain disease than brain injury, although diffuse injuries are also possible, as, for example, when a blood clot breaks up in the blood stream and then ends up in many different parts of the brain. In any event, various types of brain injuries can produce stuttering behaviors (Helm, Butler, & Canter, 1980).

Both psychogenic and neurogenic stuttering share a number of characteristics, the most notable of which is that they typically do *not* contain the struggle behaviors, the pushing and forcing of air, the muscular tension, the avoidance tricks, or the behaviors designed to hide or minimize the stuttering. Because this struggle and avoidance behavior, which makes up such a large part of the developmental stuttering profile, is missing in psychogenic and neurogenic stuttering, these two forms of the disorder seem very different from the former. They are also different in another important way. All of the fluency-enhancing strategies described in Chapter 3 have little or no effect on these two special forms of stuttering. Psychogenic and neurogenic stuttering occur just as much when the speaker is talking under masking noise, choral speech, or metronomically paced speech as without these external stimuli. Individuals with these types of the disorder also stutter when they sing, and their stuttering will be less likely to adapt with repeated reading of the same material (Roth et al., 1989).

Fortunately, psychogenic and neurogenic stuttering respond rather well to treatment. The resistance and paradox that are so common in developmental stuttering are absent, and the disorder can be dealt with in a much more straightforward way than developmental stuttering. Conversion-reaction stuttering can be treated by resolving the basic underlying conflict in the same way that aphonia, deafness, or other conversion reactions are treated. Posttraumatic-stress stuttering seems to be more difficult to treat.

Current Theories of Stuttering

In this section, a more detailed examination of stuttering will be presented. In an earlier chapter, we set aside the possibilities that stuttering is a language disorder, a disorder of voicing, or a psychoemotional disturbance. Now it can be seen that, under certain specific conditions, stuttering can be a psychoemotional disturbance, but this is quite rare. Most persons who stutter are neither more nor less neurotic than the rest of us.

Stuttering and Speech Motor Control

Contemporary theory about stuttering can be dated from an article by Zimmermann (1980). Zimmermann described stuttering as a disorder of movement, that is, what was difficult for persons who stuttered to do was move the speech mechanism during the act of speech. An obvious question is "Why only the speech mechanism?" The answer seems to be that the movements people make to produce the sounds of speech are unique in several respects—they are semiautomatic, as described earlier; they are very rapid and precise, somewhat more so than the movements of typing or playing a musical instrument; and they are organized by the brain in such a way that the speaker is able to produce a long series of movements temporally and spatially coordinated with each other. The latter characteristic is accomplished via the motor program, a set of "instructions" that the brain devises and then sends as a unit to the more peripheral structures for execution. The program is "written" first, to organize the movements of a rather lengthy sequence, perhaps a clause, then a signal to "execute" is sent that allows the sequence to be produced without further thought (Levelt, 1989).

Zimmermann (1980) proposed that this speech motor-control mechanism was disrupted in people who stuttered so that they were unable to automatically execute a written program. He suggested specifically that the difficulty these individuals had was located in the interface between these two aspects of motor control. This specificity allowed him to argue that the problem was physiologically located at the motoneuron pool, where a host of variables come together to influence the final form of the executed utterance. Thus, the speech of a person who stuttered could be influenced by events located in the central nervous system, such as a memory of difficulty talking in a particular situation, or they could also be influenced by external events that change the way a person talks, such as the fluency-enhancing conditions mentioned earlier. This theory offered a powerful explanation in that it explained both the general emotional effects, such as more stuttering when anxious or excited, and the more peripheral effects, such as less stuttering when talking more slowly. It also allowed for the learning processes that seem almost certainly to play a major role in the development of word, listener, and situation fears, and the myriad avoidance behaviors that people who stutter acquire.

Smith (1989) published the results of some research that seems to back up Zimmermann's ideas. Smith found that people who stutter have a tendency to have a rhythmic tremor deep within the muscles that does not influence the movement of the larger muscles. This tremor seems to be present at all times, although it would naturally increase in amplitude during times of stress, time pressure, and so forth, when stuttering would be more likely to occur. Although present in all muscles, this latent tremor might very well influence only the speech muscles because they are smaller and more rapid and precise in their movements than virtually all other muscles in the body.

Stuttering and Increased Levels of Muscle Activity

Van Lieshout, Peters, Starkweather, and Hulstijn (1993) published a study demonstrating that people who stutter tend to speak with elevated muscle tension. These authors asked a group of people who stutter and a group of people who do not to say a sentence that begins with a word for which lip-rounding is required. At the same time, they measured the level of activity in the muscles that perform the lip-rounding gesture. They found that the individuals who stutter used more muscle activity—that is, there was more muscle tension—for the same gesture than did the nonstuttering peers. Not only that, but this extra muscle activity persisted in the former for the duration of the sentence, even though no more lip-rounding was required in the sentence. In the nonstuttering peer group, the muscle activity returned to a lower level much sooner after the gesture was completed. The data for this study are shown in Figure 4.2. Of course, it is unlikely that this is true only for the lip muscles, but it is most probably true for all the muscles involved in speech movements. It thus seems as though when people who stutter talk, they use an abnormally tense musculature and that this persists long after the gesture that triggered it was performed. Consequently, individuals who stutter are likely to be talking with an abnormally tense speech mechanism whenever they talk, or at least once a specific gesture has triggered the tension.

Starkweather (1995b) described a "simple theory" of stuttering that accentuates the role of excessive muscle tension during the production of speech. It follows, and fits well with, the ideas of

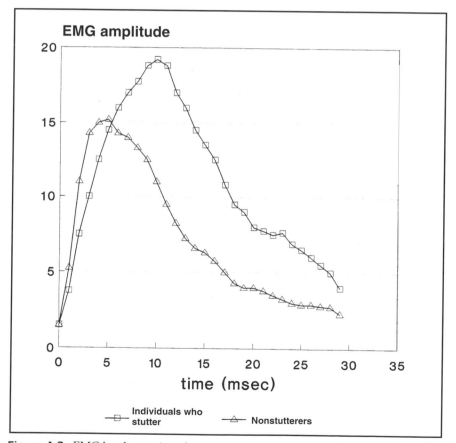

Figure 4.2. EMG level over time during a speech gesture. From "Physiological Differences between Stutterers and Nonstutterers in Perceptually Fluent Speech: EMG Amplitude and Duration," by P. H. H. M. van Lieshout, H. F. M. Peters, C. W. Starkweather, and W. Hulstijn, 1993, *Journal of Speech and Hearing Research, 36,* 55–63. Copyright 1993 by the *Journal of Speech and Hearing Research.* Reprinted with permission.

Zimmermann (1980) and Smith (1989). This theory is simple in that it does not attempt to explain the etiology of the disorder but instead calls attention to the fact that at the moment the stuttering behavior occurs, or just before it, there is excessive muscle tension. Such tension can explain most of the phenomena of stuttering, although in a few cases additional research is needed to test the theory with regard to certain specific stuttering phenomena.

Smith (1995) reviewed the literature on muscle activity level and concluded that there was little evidence of increased muscle activity during stuttering. The articles reviewed, however, consisted of studies in which the authors failed to find a statistically significant difference. Muscle activity levels are difficult to observe, particularly when a narrow time window is used, and it is not surprising that there were a number of negative results. When significant amounts of time are observed, it seems both logical and empirically verified that the extraneous behavior of stuttering is accompanied by higher levels of muscle activity.

Stuttering and Involuntary Failure of Synergy

Perkins, Kent, and Curlee (1991) also published a theory that may be summarized as stating that stuttering is a failure of motor control and prosody to synergize. The prosodic elements of speech—syllable stress and the changing melody of the voice—are related to stuttering in important ways. Nearly all stuttering behaviors occur on stressed syllables, and most individuals who can speak with greater fluency if they alter the pitch of their voice in some way—higher, lower, monotone, or excessively melodious. Without going into great detail, this theory relies heavily on the idea that stuttering is an involuntary behavior, that is, something that people who stutter do not do intentionally but rather that just happens to them. Certainly these individuals do say that they feel that the stuttering behavior is not something they do intentionally. It feels completely involuntary. This could be said about many aspects of fluent speech production, however. Imagine, for example, trying to alter one's phonologic structure for a day, such as saying /f/ wherever /s/ belonged. It would be extremely difficult to do, as difficult, one would suppose, as it would be to talk without stuttering. In addition, the normal nonfluencies of people who do not stutter are also involuntary. No one intends to say "um" or to start a sentence, stop, and then start all over again. Indeed the nonfluencies of speakers who do not stutter seem to be every bit as involuntary as those of individuals who stutter. The only difference is that the stuttering behaviors last much longer, so that there is more opportunity for the individual to feel out of control, as he or she certainly is. However, the person who does not stutter also feels out of control, just for a briefer period of time.

Stuttering and Anxiety

At this stage in the development of stuttering theory, it is widely accepted that anxiety plays little or no role in the etiology of stuttering. H. F. M. Peters and Hulstijn (1984) compared those who stuttered and those who did not before and after a speech task. They found no difference between the two groups before the task, but they did find a difference afterward, suggesting that anxiety did not contribute to the occurrence of stuttering, but that stuttering may well contribute to the occurrence of anxiety. Of course, it is always difficult to separate cause and effect, and the fact that most people who stutter report feelings of fear when they exhibit the behavior could well be simply that they know they are going to stutter and, therefore, that they are going to be embarrassed or ashamed. The negative feelings would be expected as a consequence of the disorder.

There is another possibility. People who stutter do not typically report heavy anxiety or massive, long-lasting feelings of fear. Instead, they report feeling a spike of fear just before they stutter. This is so common a comment that it might be taken to be almost universal. How can this be reconciled with the Peters and Hulstijn report of no difference between the two groups before a speech task? It may be that the ability to identify accurately such a brief spike of fear is lacking. It would not be present before the general speech act and yet appear during speech just before the word that ends up being produced with stuttering. More research with tools designed to capture such a brief emotional spike seems required.

Criteria for a Theory of Stuttering

Any theory of stuttering should be able to explain a number of facts. These facts, described earlier, are as follows:

1. Many more males stutter than do females;

2. People who stutter are slower in moving the speech mechanism than those who do not;

3. Certain externally imposed conditions—slower rate, DAF, FAF, choral speech, and so forth—promote fluency;

4. There is very little stuttering among the deaf;

5. Stuttering is distributed in families according to a genetically determined pattern; and

6. Stuttering occurs in some situations (words, listeners) more than in others in a given individual.

In addition, a theory of stuttering should explain how the disorder can develop in children, and it should make a clear distinction between the normal nonfluencies of individuals who do not stutter and the behaviors of those who do. Perkins et al.'s (1991) theory seems not to differentiate between normal nonfluencies and stuttering behaviors. Theories of speech motor control, such as those of Zimmermann (1980), seem to do so by looking at the level of movement. It is the movements that are abnormal, and, thus, it seems likely that the muscle activity underlying the movements may also be abnormal. It is important to remember, however, that these are not theories of etiology. They address simply how to describe the disorder, not what causes it.

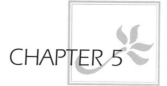

CHAPTER 5

Evaluation

E valuation is a two-way street. The clinician is evaluating the client and his or her disorder, and the client is evaluating the clinician with regard to competence, compatibility, and cost. This is most appropriate because as therapy moves forward both client and clinician will be changed by their interaction. In the case of very seasoned clinicians, the client will surely change more than the clinician, but in the case of neophyte clinicians, it could well be the other way around.

In evaluating or assessing a person who stutters, a speech clinician attempts to obtain sufficient information to describe the problem as it presents itself. This description needs to distinguish between those aspects of the disorder that are objectively observable and those that are a matter of opinion. It also must describe and quantify accurately, where possible.

In evaluating a clinician, a client will want to determine if the person is qualified to perform the task, if he or she understands the disorder and the person who has it, and if that professional listens well. In addition, the client will want to find out if the clinician can make a prognosis of outcome and estimate how long therapy will last. There will be times when the clinician cannot answer these last two questions, and clients will need to accept that. There can be no guarantee of successful treatment; providing such a guarantee is a violation of the Code of Ethics of ASHA. If a client hears such a guarantee or something that sounds like one, they should be suspicious of the clinician's qualifications. Clinicians can, however, give information about the successes they may have had with previous clients. Clients will find it useful to make contact with previous clients, although the clinician will not be able to divulge their names until they have given permission. Potential clients reading this book will find it helpful to read the

Guidelines for Practice in Stuttering Treatment, which is reprinted in its entirety in Appendix A. It includes a list of competencies that clinicians treating persons who stutter ought to have.

Case History

The history of the client's disorder, from its beginning to the present, is important for the purpose of determining, insofar as is possible, the influences on the person's stuttering behavior. In addition, it is important to reach an understanding about the larger problem(s) created by the disorder in the person's life. To do this, the clinician requires some general information about the person—level of education, medical history, social and family life. This gives the clinician information not only about the client, but also about how, when, how often, where, and for what purposes he or she uses speech. This wider context comes together in the case history.

Providing Information

Clinicians also provide information at the time of the assessment, and clients should feel comfortable about asking questions. Adults with children who stutter and adults who stutter themselves have many questions when they come to see the speech clinician. Some of these questions can be deferred until a more complete description of the disorder is obtained, but often the clinician will provide general information about the disorder at the time of the initial meeting. Clinicians will typically talk to parents about the genetic aspect of stuttering—explaining to them what is known and what is not known about the tendency for stuttering to run in families. Giving information about the disorder and about treatment to clients and parents of clients is an important first step in overcoming a sense of helplessness that many clients have when they first seek the help of a speech clinician.

It is also helpful at this time for clients to learn that stuttering, like tooth decay, is the kind of problem that should be checked on from time to time. There is a tendency for the disorder to reoccur, usually slowly insinuating itself back into the person's speech. Although this tendency is clearly present in adults, it is either very much smaller or completely absent in preschool children. When therapy is finally terminated, clients should expect to come back from time to time to make sure that the gains made previously have not eroded.

Providing Support

Clinicians also begin to offer support at the time of the initial evaluation. The goal of all treatment is to support the client in his or her recovery without creating a dependency on the clinician. Clients are told from the beginning that recovery from stuttering involves some self-confrontation and hard work. At the same time, most clients benefit from treatment, so it is appropriate to convey the idea that treatment will be useful. Many clients will ask if there is a cure. The answer to this question is complex. The word cure is not appropriate; stuttering is not a disease. As discussed in this text, it is highly individualized; therefore, treatment must also be individualized. There is no single technique. It might be more appropriate to ask "Do people recover from stuttering?" The only difficulty with this question is the definition of recovery. Most clients have been trying hard for a long time to be more fluent, that is, free from stuttering. In many cases, the effort they put into trying to talk without stuttering is the main problem. As was discussed in Chapter 2, true fluency is more than simply the absence of stuttering; it is the ability to talk at a normal rate with normal speech and movement and minimal muscular and mental effort (Starkweather, 1987). The clinician whose primary goal in treatment is to have clients speak without stuttering is working from the same attitude and perspective that has made life so difficult for the client. The main goal of therapy should be a feeling of freedom in speaking, of talking without the extra burdens that stuttering and the attempts to control stuttering can create. Out of this recovery an easiness of speech, that is, true "freedom of speech," can develop.

Evaluation of Fluency

In evaluating the person's fluency, the clinician measures three aspects: speech rate, articulatory rate, and speech continuity. The rate at which the person is able to produce words, including all the time taken up by pauses, hesitations, and dysfluencies, is simply the total number of syllables[1] divided by the total number of seconds during which the person was talking. This speech rate is a general descriptor of a person's ability to produce information within a period of time.

It is also useful to measure the person's articulatory rate, that is, the number of syllables per second that the person produces when speech is fluent. This is done by removing all the time taken up by stuttering behaviors, or other forms of dysfluency, and using the residual time as the denominator. Articulatory rate gives the clinician some sense of the person's speech motor ability. It should be noted that this measure can be contaminated by attempts to talk slowly, which may have been discovered by the client or taught as a treatment.

The continuity of speech is also assessed. As mentioned earlier, continuity is the extent to which speech flows along without interruption by extraneous, that is, unintended elements such as repetitions, filled pauses and broken words. It is relatively easy to discern what the person would have said had these extraneous elements not been present (Levelt, 1989). This intended utterance is the starting point in assessing continuity. It permits the separation of the extraneous elements, or discontinuities, from the intention. These elements can then be counted, categorized, and measured for duration. Depending on need, there are two ways to do this. For "quick-and-dirty" estimates, a simple frequency count of discontinuities can be performed. The busy clinician who has only limited time may have to settle for this. A better, more complete, measure of the person's level of continuity can be obtained by summing the durations of all discontinuities and dividing this sum by the duration of the complete utterance, including discontinuities. This provides the clinician with the percentage of discontinuous speech time (PDST), and is a more complete account of the person's level of speech continuity. Although a valid and reliable description of speech continuity, the PDST has one disadvantage as a clinical tool—it includes time taken up by normal nonfluencies, which people who stutter also have, as well as time taken up by stuttering behaviors. However, Ingham and Cordes, (1992), Young (1984), and others have shown that this distinction cannot be reliably made in any case. Because all speakers have a certain baseline level of discontinuity, there seems to be no point in trying to make the distinction (see Figure 5.1 for a worked example).

---

[1]Words are also sometimes used, but syllables are slightly more accurate.

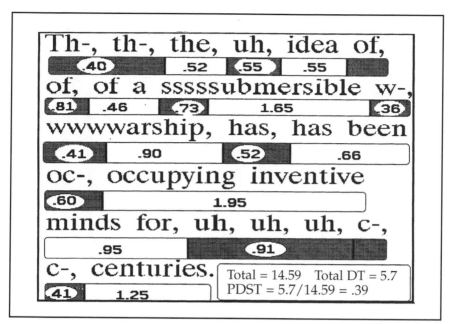

Figure 5.1. A worked example of the calculation for PDST.

It is important to remember that fluency varies over time and from situation to situation. This implies that the measures made of a sample taken in the clinic may not be representative of the person's speech in everyday life. Repeated samples taken from a variety of real-life situations can be gathered and compared with the sample taken during the initial evaluation. In addition, the client should be asked if the obtained sample is typical of his or her speech in other circumstances. The clinician should make a note of any discrepancies, and their direction, in the final report.

Defensive reactions also need to be assessed. If they occupy time, they will be included in the PDST, but if they do not occupy time (an accompanying hand gesture, or rapid eye-blinking, for example), they need to be further described. The exact nature of the secondary reactions often needs to be described in detail because these reactions can be quite individual. Finally, the clinician should make some attempt to determine how successful the client is in avoiding stuttering because a successful avoider will have a correspondingly reduced count of overt stuttering. This can be approximated by asking the person to try as hard as they can not to stutter. Instructions to "just go ahead and stutter as much as you like"—in essence, giving "permission" to stutter—can provide some insight into this variable, although they are usually difficult for clients to follow because the habit of avoidance may be very strong and the prohibition against stuttering very powerful. The development of a reliable tool for determining the successfulness of defensive reactions in reducing the frequency of overt stuttering behaviors is an important research need.

Evaluation of Capacities

Motor Capacities

In both children and adults, the best indicator of speech motor skill is articulatory rate. How quickly is the person able to produce syllables? Evidence suggests that we all talk nearly (but not quite) as fast as we can and that we hate to slow down (Tiffany, 1980). This drive to communicate at a fast pace probably even plays a role in the emotional reactions that speakers and listeners alike have to the time-consuming extraneous behaviors of stuttering. Measures of speech motor skill that are independent of fluency are not yet available, although a research effort is under way (H. F. M. Peters, Hulstijn, & van Lieshout, 1995).

Linguistic Capacities

Children who stutter or are at risk for stuttering are tested for their linguistic knowledge and performance. Knowledge of syntax, semantics, pragmatics, and phonology allows children to express complex thoughts and feelings in a more adult way; however, at the same time these linguistic areas make substantial demands on the child's capacity for producing syllables. Speech is both a linguistic and a motor act, and it has been demonstrated that increased difficulty in one can diminish performance in the other (Kinsbourne & Hicks, 1978). The child who knows longer words wants to use them, and his or her parents delight in it, which encourages the child. Similarly, the child who knows how to formulate long, complex sentences will do so to communicate the complex ideas he or she has. The child whose phonological knowledge permits the pronunciation of new, unfamiliar words may still not be able to make the necessary combination of coordinated movements needed to utter them. And the child whose pragmatic knowledge permits interactions that are more socially acceptable and mature may not have the emotional maturity with which to do so. This linguistic knowledge makes it a little more difficult for the child who stutters or is at risk for stuttering to produce the sentences he or she knows.

On the other hand, linguistic performance—the finding of words, the construction of sentences, the utterance of socially appropriate interactions, and the generation of phonologically correct syllables—is a capacity. These components that make up linguistic performance serve fluency. The child who cannot find words or construct sentences quickly, or who cannot easily produce a complex syllable, gives up some time to the process; the child who feels uncomfortable in an ambiguous or complex social situation will be more hesitant than the child who has more sophisticated pragmatic skills. These skills promote fluency, and their relative lack diminishes a child's capacity to speak quickly and easily.

In most adults, both knowledge and use of language will be well formed and thus do not hinder fluent communication. Occasionally, however, an adult with poor word-finding or sentence-formulation skills, or a lack of practice in social situations (often as a result of having stuttered for many years), will find that these problems contribute to reduced fluency. More often, diminished linguistic capacity contributes to the development of stuttering, which becomes more "hardwired" as the child grows and plasticity of development is reduced (Brauth, Hall, & Dooling, 1991; Ludlow, 1996). Eventually the child may develop the capacities for fluency that his or her environment requires, but the pattern of speaking with struggle and forcing, accompanied by repetition, prolongation, blockage, and hesitation, has become entrenched as a part of the child's approach to, and execution of, speech. Change becomes more difficult.

Emotional Capacities

An evaluation of a child or adult's emotional capacities for fluency cannot objectively be made. Most clinicians, however, are able to assess a child's general level of emotional maturity by noting such behavioral events as the ease or difficulty with which the child separates from the parent, the child's level of "shyness," and so forth. It frequently is helpful to ask the parents to give some adjectives that they would use to describe their child. When the parent uses words such as nervous, high strung, intense, or sensitive, the clinician will know that he or she should consider the child's emotional maturity as possibly being lower than is typical for that age group.

Adults also vary in the extent to which they can handle emotional circumstances. Clinicians will want to know how nervous, angry, depressed, or contented an adult client is. There are no objective tests for these characteristics that can be easily used in the speech therapy setting, and many tests in this area can be administered only by certified psychotherapists. In most cases of stuttering it is not necessary to make such a formal assessment, and, as therapy continues, the clinician will get to know the client well enough to make an informal assessment that is sufficient. It should be noted that in some cases emotional factors play a more important role, and a referral to a qualified psychologist may be useful. The decision to refer for psychological evaluation should be made on a case-by-case basis, and it is best made jointly with the client. If the information that such an evaluation would provide will be helpful in planning or executing therapy, then the clinician and client together ought to be able to see the value of it.

As a rule, psychoemotional evaluation of adults is not taken as a means to uncover etiological factors for stuttering, but rather to identify client characteristics that need to be considered in planning or carrying out a program of recovery. In most cases, stuttering has a substantial, if not profound, impact on the person's confidence, sociability, anxiety level, identity, shame, and happiness. In addition, people who stutter are subject to all the rest of life's difficulties and traumas. A dysfunctional family background, with or without alcoholism or addiction of some other kind, will make it all the more difficult to cope with a stuttering problem. Both client and clinician need to know about any such background that might be relevant to the client. Furthermore, when real emotional problems exist, they will usually have an impact on the client's stuttering in some important ways, such as influencing the behaviors themselves, the circumstances under which they occur, the type and extent of struggle and avoidance reactions, and many other aspects.

Cognitive Capacities

As with emotional capacities, a child's level of cognitive development is assessed informally. The content and style of the child's play are excellent indicators of cognitive level. It is also useful to ask the client questions about speech to gauge his or her level of understanding regarding the process and his or her metalinguistic skill in describing it.

It is helpful to find out what the adult client knows and believes about stuttering. Here, too, the client's history of the problem will provide substantial insights. Every individual who stutters has a story to tell of how he or she came to be that person. This story is the single most important piece of diagnostic information the clinician can obtain because it determines many elements of the client's perceptions, beliefs, and attitudes toward stuttering, toward speech, and toward socialization in general.

Evaluating the Environment

A significant change in the past 15 years has been the systematic evaluation and measurement of the *communicative environment* of a person who stutters. This term refers to any stimuli—events or ongoing characteristics—that can have an impact on a person's fluency level. The communicative environment can be either demanding or facilitating of fluency. In preschool children, an important source of these stimuli is the communicative behavior (verbal and nonverbal) of the child's parents and siblings, playschool teachers, babysitters, nannies, and so forth. The general milieu also is important, particularly with regard to the important emotional effects—excitement and anxiety—and to the always important influence of time pressure.

As children approach school age, the power of these external environmental influences begins to diminish as the child takes on or internalizes the reactions of significant adults. By the time he or she enters school, the influence of adults has waned considerably and the importance of peer evaluation has risen substantially. Toward the end of school life, self-evaluation starts to replace peer evaluation. Consequently, by the time a person who stutters has reached adulthood, the internal environment is as important as the external one.

There are four aspects of the internal and external environments that need to be evaluated. These four areas correspond to the four areas of skill, or capacities, that any person brings to the act of talking: motor, language, socioemotional, and cognitive abilities that the person uses in producing fluent speech. Similarly, the communicative environment may be demanding or facilitating of fluency in each of these four skill areas.

Influence on the Motor System

In order to produce fluent speech, individuals need to move the various parts of the vocal tract quickly and smoothly so that long strings of intelligible syllables can be continuously and rapidly produced. The speed and smoothness of these movements are components of fluency. The accuracy of these movements, although obviously vital for the intelligibility of speech, is not a capacity for fluency, but a demand, as shall momentarily be shown.

A number of environmental factors can challenge or facilitate a person's speech motor skills. First and foremost are any environmental events that require the person to move the speech mechanism more rapidly. The more rapidly a series of speech movements are made, the more elevated the activity in the muscles producing those movements (Armson, 1991). Because many of the speech muscles are organized into antagonistic sets, such that a contraction of one muscle requires a simultaneous relaxed extension of another, rapid movements increase the extent of overlap of antagonistic muscle activities, causing the antagonistic muscles momentarily to pull against each other. In other words, with increasing velocity of movements, there is a tendency for an increase in the amount of time antagonistic muscles will be simultaneously co-contracting. The simultaneous co-contraction of antagonistic muscles increases the overall level of stiffness in the system and the general level of effort that is required for all movements. Stiff systems do not move quickly or easily. At a certain threshold of stiffness, systems tend to go into oscillation or tremor.

Fortunately, for most speakers there is a kind of safety valve. As speech gets faster, it is possible to keep muscles from getting too tense by reducing the precision of articulatory placement and by overlapping certain gestures in time. This strategy, called *undershoot* or *coarticulation,* makes it possible to increase the rate of syllable production without increasing the stiffness of the mechanism. In fact, it is possible to reduce muscle activity levels while keeping rate constant or even increase it a little, via the same strategy. This coping mechanism has been discovered and employed by some people who stutter.

Unfortunately, there is a negative consequence—the precision of articulation deteriorates. However, because speech is a highly redundant system, a substantial decrease in the precision of articulatory placement, although it reduces intelligibility, can allow the speaker to still communicate effectively.

De Nil and Brutten (1988) discovered that people who stutter cannot use coarticulatory undershoot as a strategy for increasing rate as well as peers who do not stutter. This may be a physiological difference (a lower capacity), but it may also be an environmental one (a higher demand). Many people who stutter report having been taught the importance of clear, carefully articulated speech and the general tendency toward perfectionism that some of these individuals have (Amster, 1995) may suggest a more demanding environment.

Time Pressure

In any event, the clinician evaluates the person's environment for characteristics that may tend to increase motivation to talk faster. It is important to note that the question is not whether the person actually does talk faster, because the attempt to talk faster can produce speech that is slower as a result of the build-up of muscle tension described above and because of time-occupying slips, stumbles, or stutters that additional tension produces. The important question is whether the internal or external environments are such that the person is induced to talk faster.

Several factors induce people to talk faster; time pressure is the most obvious. When parents or siblings, babysitters, or any other significant person in a child's environment talks more rapidly than the child, there is some pressure through vicarious conditioning (modeling) and the well-known "convergence" effects for the child to try to speed up to match the other speaker's rate. Because adults in general tend to talk faster than do children, there is always some of this time pressure on children.

Measuring the speech rate of the parents and other significant speakers in the child's environment and then comparing these rates to that of the child provides an index of the amount of time pressure the child may be receiving. Although there are no established norms for the difference between adult and child speech rates, making it impossible to identify a specific number above which parents' speech rate could be characterized as demanding, the clinician who takes this measure at intake has an objective way to assess progress in the reduction of time pressure.

In adults, the role played by the speech rate of listeners should be assessed. Many adults who stutter report that it is much more difficult to talk to someone who is a rapid speaker. Unfortunately, it is also often the case that speakers will speed up when they talk to a person who stutters. The extra time that the stuttering takes up puts both the person who stutters and the conversational partner under increased time pressure.

Another measurable source of time pressure is the length of sentences (utterances) the person produces. It has been shown that longer utterances are spoken more quickly, both in adults and in children (Amster, 1984; Malecot, Johnston, & Kizziar, 1972). It is not clear whether this relationship between utterance length and speech rate is attributable to respiratory requirements or some perceived standard of information flow (Starkweather, 1987), and it is generally rather difficult to achieve a pervasive reduction in utterance length. Nevertheless, the measure is useful in providing an overall picture of the amount of time pressure the person may be under.

The remaining sources of time pressures are (a) a generally rushed household, (b) the frequent occurrence of social situations in which time pressure is a notable feature (e.g., ordering in a restaurant with a line of customers behind you), and (c) saying one's name or answering the telephone. These are difficult to quantify. Despite this, they still should be evaluated as part of the assessment procedure, although the information obtained in the assessment will be unquantified verbal descriptions, making it relatively less useful in measuring progress than more quantifiable measures.

Other Demands on Motor Performance

There is always a trading relationship between movement precision and movement speed. The faster one tries to perform an act, the more difficult it is to perform it accurately. Alternatively, the more precisely one must perform an act, the more time it will need. The same is true for speech. When the circumstances require that a word or sentence be said more precisely, it places a demand on the speech motor system. Sometimes the requirement to say something very clearly results in a slower rate that is completely acceptable. As a result, fluency may increase. If there is some time pressure in addition to a requirement for precision, however, fluency may deteriorate. For example, under noisy circumstances most adults who stutter are more fluent. One explanation for this is that speech is slower under noise, an aspect of the well-known Lombard Effect. On the other hand, people who stutter usually stutter more when asked to repeat themselves in a normal conversation by a listener who asks "What?" (Longhurst & Siegel,

1973). This is probably because the demand for precision has increased while the time pressure has remained the same or even increased. Similarly, when a child who stutters grows up in a family where precision of articulation is valued, this value may become part of the person's internal environment as an adult and place a demand for precision during a wide variety of social circumstances.

Demands on the Linguistic System

In order to produce appropriately long strings of syllables that are smoothly joined and produced at a normally rapid rate, the child must be able to formulate the sentences he or she wants to say so that when they occur they will be grammatical. In addition, the child must be able to retrieve from his or her lexicon the words that are appropriate to the intended meaning. Both sentence formulation and word-finding occupy time, and when they are difficult for the person, they may occupy a considerable amount of time. Sentence formulation becomes highly automatic in adults, but sometimes this is a disadvantage. When word substitution is used habitually as an avoidance behavior from an early age, the process of substituting words can become an aspect of sentence formulation. The senior author has seen numerous clients whose word substitution was far too automatic for them to be aware of it, and the junior author has had personal experience with this phenomenon. Thus, word finding for both children and adults, and sentence formulation for children, are skills or capacities for fluency, and environmental events or features that make word finding and sentence formulation more difficult are demands on fluency. Consequently, when the topic of a conversation involves words and structures of this demanding kind, it is to be expected that more stuttering will occur.

The Concept of Interference

During speech production, all four of the areas just mentioned are simultaneously active. Speech production is always a motoric, linguistic, socioemotional, and cognitive act. When any one of these areas is stressed, it may interfere with the functioning of the other areas. Kinsbourne and Hicks (1978) showed the extent of this interference effect in experiments demonstrating that people were less able to perform coordinated motor acts while they were talking. Furthermore, the extent of the interference was proportional to the distance between the two areas of the brain being used. It seems unlikely that such interference is limited only to language activity with motor performance (Starkweather, 1991). It has also been shown that emotional demands can interfere with motor performance (Hill, 1954). For example, most of us have experienced the interference effect of cognitive functioning on language (the difficulty of verbalizing a really complicated thought) or emotional demands on cognition ("I can't think about that right now; I am too upset"). As far as fluency is concerned, it is probably most important to note that conditions requiring more difficult cognitive, emotional, or linguistic functioning can interfere with motor performance.

It may be argued with some legitimacy that the ability to produce fluent speech is, in and of itself, an ability to syngergize these four areas of function. It seems likely, in fact, that the human speech-production mechanism (including linguistic functioning) has been genetically selected in a way that makes such synergies possible. This argument does not, it seems to us, detract from the possibility that, as the difficulty of one element of this synergistic system is increased, the functioning of another element may be compromised. In fact, it seems more likely that, given the close functional ties that such a synergistic view implies, the probability of interference of one element by another is increased rather than diminished.

Sentence Formulation

With the concept of interference in hand, we can now consider what aspects of a person's environment make it more difficult (and this means specifically more time consuming) for him or her to formulate sentences and find words. First, and most obvious, if the person is trying to formulate sentences that are syntactically more complex, the formulation process should be more difficult and more time consuming. But how much time does sentence formulation require? Not much is known about this (Levelt, 1989), and the development of an understanding of it is made more complex by the fact that sentence formulation takes place simultaneously for the most part with other functions, and, of course, it is a process that is not directly observable. Although it seems intuitively appealing to assume that more complex sentences are more time demanding than simpler ones, there are no data that specify how much actual time is involved. It remains possible that the formulation of more complex sentences may demand more time, but it may not demand enough time to matter insofar as the fluency of speech production is concerned. It may, however, interfere with motor processes in a way that is demanding of time.

We do know, of course, that both normal nonfluencies and stuttering behaviors are more likely to occur when material is syntactically more complex (Cecconi, Hood, & Tucker, 1977; Gordon, Luper, & Peterson, 1986), and, at least in the case of normal nonfluencies, it is actually sentence formulation that is responsible (Gordon & Peterson, 1982).

In spite of these uncertainties, it is surely desirable for speech clinicians evaluating the environments of preschool or school-age children at risk for chronic stuttering, or in the early stages of stuttering, to obtain some measures of the child's language performance, including syntactic complexity. Because of the uncertain relationship between this measure and fluency, it seems wise not to devote an unusual amount of time to the measure but to use one of the several "quick-and-dirty" estimates. In addition, because of the possibility of additional difficulty in sentence formulation that such complexity may create, when developing a child's treatment plan one should consider the possibility that sentence formulation may interfere with the motoric planning or execution of syllable production. It should also be noted that because complex sentences tend to be longer, and longer sentences spoken more quickly, the effect on motor execution may be via this indirect route, rather than directly via sentence formulation itself.

It seems unlikely that the complexity of the parents' language influences the complexity of the child's, but it *is* likely that the *amount* of talking that the parents do can accelerate the child's language development, in some cases well beyond the child's motoric capacity to produce long, rapid utterances. Consequently, a measure of parental talking time is a quantifiable index of the amount of language stimulation the preschool child receives. Language overstimulation (see the section on reducing demands on the motor system in Chapter 6) is one of the ways stuttering can develop.

For adults, it is sufficient simply to see if there is a relationship between the complexity of the sentence a person is trying to say and the likelihood that stuttering will occur on the sentence. Many people who stutter will be aware of such a relationship, but there are some who will demonstrate the relationship without being aware of it.

Word Finding

Word finding is another matter. In this case it is known—usually from personal experience as well as from research literature—that the process of finding a word can occupy amounts of time that, in the fleeting world of speech production, are quite significant. Some children and adults have specific deficits of word finding that in themselves detract from fluency. In the case of children also at risk for developing a chronic stuttering problem, these deficits can increase demands for fluency by increasing the time the child needs for speech production. In addition, in children for whom fluency is not a challenge, environmental events that increase word-finding difficulty will add time to speech production and also interfere indirectly with the motor process of speech production.

As with syntactic complexity, it is the person's knowledge of long, relatively infrequently used words that can challenge his or her capacity for fluency. Longer and less frequently used words are far more likely to be stuttered than shorter, more common ones (Soderberg, 1966). Some measure of vocabulary or semantic diversity thus seems appropriate. The person with a more extensive vocabulary who makes full use of the semantic diversity that such a vocabulary offers is producing utterances containing words that, because of their relative rarity and length, are more evocative of pauses, hesitations, and pathological stuttering behaviors. In addition, longer words tend to be spoken more quickly than shorter ones (van Lieshout et al., 1995), although the effect is relatively small.

Demands on Socioemotional Functioning

The relationship between emotion and stuttering is curiously ambivalent. On the one hand, nearly all people who stutter report that the problem is associated with fear. They feel afraid that they will be embarrassed or humiliated; that they will become so stuck that they cannot get moving again; that listeners will think them stupid, crazy, or "nervous"; or, in many cases, that they will have to reveal their stuttering. Many of these individuals also fear the tendency of listeners to look away or in some other way stop listening. Like any other person in the act of communicating, they want to be heard, and fear that their ideas will not be received if they are not heard. All of these fears can make stuttering more severe.

On the other hand, research (H. F. M. Peters & Hulstijn, 1984) has tended to show that both individuals who stutter and those who do not are not much different in their anxiety levels before they begin to talk. They become different in this way after they talk, suggesting that the fears of people who stutter are created by the stuttering, rather than the other way around. It seems to us, however, that the issue of fear causing stuttering has not yet been fully resolved. It seems likely, that, in the very high speed of ongoing speech production, a spike of fear or panic could occur that would have a direct and substantial, although momentary, influence on the person's ability to move smoothly and quickly in order to produce syllables. Such a brief spike of fear would not be detectable by any but the most refined physiological monitoring system. Such systems have not been used in the experiments on stuttering and fear. These spikes of fear, which sound very similar to what people who stutter report, have not yet been assessed. It thus is possible that there is a causative influence of fear on speech production that has not been tested or observed.

Illustrative of the complexity of the relationship between emotion and stuttering is the following quotation from a posting on the Internet.

> Refusing to own up that stuttering hurts has implications for therapy and a lot of other stuff. For me (at least as a kid) going to therapy was an admission that there was something wrong with me. Having to practice my speech techniques was even worse. I could never practice. I'd start doing my vowel exercises and I'd start to cry. Doing those vowels meant admitting to myself that I had a handicap. That I was defective, that I wasn't "normal" like everyone else. Rather than deal with the pain of that admission, I stopped practicing. Which allowed me to stop crying, which allowed me to go outside and play with my friends, which allowed me to be happy and feel good about myself. This . . . attitude . . . made me feel good at that time. There [was] a positive aspect to it. I did live a "normal" boy's life and learn skills that gave me confidence in every other area of my life. I never felt as if I had a disability or that I was a victim of anything.
>
> But there is a down side. Denial ultimately strikes back. Because of my strong ego I resisted change in the one area where I needed most to change. In my speech. Because to accept help meant acknowledging that I had a weakness, that I was in need of repair. It never bothered me much when people asked me about my stuttering. . . . Similarly, I've always been able to deal with stuttering in

public even if people tittered or laughed. I could grin and bear it. The pain of my embarrassment was shortlived and didn't cut very deep. . . . What's worse for me is having someone breach my secret, catch on to the fact of what I most want to deny—that my stuttering does cause me pain.

An example: I'm in the movies as a teenager watching a British comedy in which one of the characters stutters badly. The first time this character stutters on screen, the friend I was with steals a sneaky look at me to see how I'm reacting to the guy on screen stuttering. Correctly, she understands that I will identify with his stuttering and, having a lively curiosity, she want to see how I react. Had I been able, then, to confront my feelings about my stuttering, I could have (at the end of the movie) engaged her in a friendship-bonding conversation about stuttering, identity, feelings, etc.—how I felt about seeing someone stuttering on screen. The thought of that possibility went through my mind, but I was afraid to take the risk and quickly shut the door to that opening. Instead, I interpreted her glance as her wanting to see if I was as embarrassed by the portrayal as she (as I projected my feelings on to her) thought I ought to be. As for myself, I went rigid, steeling myself against any show of emotion. I wanted her to think that I took no note of the character's stuttering and did not identify with him at all—which was obviously a major lie. Nevertheless, I felt totally exposed by her glance at me, naked really, as if all my efforts to cover up my vulnerability were stripped from me. Although I often stuttered in talking to her and had no illusion that my stuttering was a secret, I could not tolerate her recognizing me and (as I interpreted it) defining me as a stutterer and nothing else. I was so wounded to be exposed. She knew my secret! Which was not that I stuttered but that I had feelings about it, that it was painful to me, that deep inside I really did believe that it represented a flaw in me, a problem.

Because of this movie, actually because of that one glance she made towards me, I withdrew from our friendship. Just dropped her. To emphasize: Not because of my stuttering, but because she knew what I refused to admit to myself: stuttering hurts. (M. Jezer, personal communication, September 21, 1995)

Preschool children, who have far less social sophistication and awareness than adults, are more likely to be frustrated than afraid as a reaction to their own stuttering. But the effects of fear of other kinds, or a more generalized anxiety, or of high levels of excitement on stuttering in the preschool child are well known and widely reported. Therefore, the clinician interested in planning therapy for the preschool child needs to assess the environment for sources of anxiety and excitement, both of which are potent disruptors of fluency in the preschool child.

An important environmental variable is the parents' level of comfort or discomfort with the topic of stuttering. Discomfort can manifest itself in a large variety of nonverbal behaviors—wincing, rolling the eyes, looking away, holding the breath, stopping all body movements until the stuttering event has passed, turning or walking away, or looking afraid or pained. Another manifestation of discomfort is the "conspiracy of silence"—just not talking about the stuttering or even acknowledging its existence. Parents who do not talk about it unwittingly deny their child parental support and comfort at a time when it is crucially needed. In addition, this pattern of parental reactions may result in a distorted perception on the part of the child concerning the extent to which people can hear and notice the stuttering behaviors. Discomfort in the parents during stuttering can also manifest itself in increasing speech rate, asking additional questions, and interrupting more frequently. All these verbal and nonverbal manifestations of discomfort send the child a strong message that stuttering is undesirable at best and shameful at worst.

As described previously, the child's knowledge of language places demands on his or her use of language and, therefore, on the ability to produce spoken words. In addition, other linguistic demands may further reduce fluency. When a bilingual child is asked to interpret for his or her parents, or when a child is asked to recite memorized passages or use speech in any nonspontaneous way, fluency level seems to decrease.

One child we knew was the only child of a couple who were troubled by a considerable amount of marital discord. Often, they would be so angry with each other that they were unable to talk to each other. At these times, they would often ask the child to speak in their place. In effect, he was playing the role of a shuttle diplomat, carrying messages back and forth between the two warring parties. At the age of 4, he was not emotionally equipped for diplomacy, particularly when it was his parents who were in such a heavy negotiation. This pattern was revealed to the clinician when she asked the mother about times when the child's stuttering was at its worst. The mother answered that it was when he was engaged in this shuttle diplomacy between her and her husband.

Another child we knew was the son of immigrants whose mastery of English was poor. Because the child had easily picked up the language of his new country in the year that he had lived there and played in the street with English-speaking playmates, on occasion he was asked to interpret for his parents. The difficulty was that these times when the parents needed an interpreter tended to be for rather serious matters, for example, when they might need to talk to a police officer, social worker, or other official. Asking the child to take on such a heavy responsibility tended to make his stuttering much worse.

These uses of language, to deliver messages or to interpret, are examples of using speech in a way that is not spontaneous. Spontaneous speech means saying what you are thinking without any concern for the form that the utterance takes. When a young child is asked to use speech in some other way—to convey the thoughts of others or to perform in some way—he or she is not speaking spontaneously. From the point of view of pragmatics, this is a more difficult task than spontaneous speech, and the ability to use speech in this nonspontaneous way is often not acquired until children are 8 or 9 years old, when they show an interest in imitating other speakers and when they become quite adept at lying.

Parents often can inadvertently make increased demands on their children for fluency through their nonverbal and verbal reactions to the child's stuttering. One of the most important areas for clinicians to assess, parental nonverbal reactions are the means by which children at risk for stuttering seem to acquire beliefs and attitudes about themselves, their speech, and their stuttering that direct them toward strategies of avoidance, denial, and struggle. Nonverbal parental reactions seem also to be the channel through which children acquire a fear of stuttering or a sense of shame because they stutter.

Clinicians can best assess nonverbal reactions of parents by making a videotape of the parents and the child playing together. Although it is necessary to inform the parents that this is being done, it rarely influences the behavior of the child, and the parents' behavior seems to be influenced mostly in the early part of the tape. Despite requests not to do so, a small number of parents do seem to try to make the child speak. This suggests to the clinician that the parents are eager to have the clinician validate their experience of the child's stuttering. It also suggests that they have not grasped the purpose of the evaluation. Both of these possibilities are significant findings. However, in most cases a reasonably valid record of the parent–child interaction can be obtained. When examined closely at a later time, parental reactions that might have gone unnoticed before can be observed, counted, and measured for duration. For later comparison and validation of change brought about by therapy concerning nonverbal reactions, the videotape is the only way to preserve aspects of the parent–child interaction that may be an important source of demands for fluency.

Perhaps the most fruitful use of such a videotape is to show it to the parents so they can see from a more objective standpoint their interaction with the child. This should not be done for the purpose of finding fault, which will only increase what is usually an already elevated sense of guilt. Elements of this interaction, including nonverbal reactions, can be described. We do not think it is wise to ask parents directly to modify their nonverbal behavior because nonverbal communicative behavior happens largely below the level of conscious awareness. Bringing it into awareness seems to make it awkward and uncomfortable. Instead, we advocate taking steps to help the parents work through the emotion that lies behind the nonverbal behavior.

Another "demand" that occurs in some families is the parents' or one parent's use of an instructional, rather than a conversational, style of interaction with the child. Although teaching is one of the things parents do, there are times when a parent, uncomfortable with genuine conversations with their child, will choose the more familiar instructional style. Often these parents are teachers who have learned that instruction is a way they can interact comfortably with children. When the instructional style is used to the exclusion of a warmer and more intimate style of conversation, the child may be missing out on some of the connectedness that should come from family life. As a result, the child's level of insecurity may be elevated, and this can have an impact on his or her general fluency level.

Although not all of these variables can be objectively measured, clinicians measure them where possible, record them when they can, and attempt to assess their influence on the person's speech. In addition, clinicians try to assess qualitatively the amount of time pressure in the home, the ambient level of anxiety and tension, the level of excitement in the person's life, and any advice that may have been given to the person that may have inadvertently increased his or her tendency to see the human social interaction mediated by speech as a treacherous place to navigate.

Demands on Cognitive Functioning

The quantity and quality of thought that go into an utterance can require a substantial amount of time, both before and during the production of it. Ideas that are complex, confusing, capable of mis-interpretation, abstract, or unusual may introduce time into the speak-er's production via hesitation, revision, or stumbling. In addition, there is also a close correspondence between language and cognition such that unusual ideas may require more words and more complex syntactical forms to explicate.

Similarly, more abstract ideas call for words that are less common and longer. Confusing or partially thought out ideas may introduce revision, as will ideas that may be misunderstood or be a source of embarrassment. Such thoughts are likely to result in substantial and sometimes multiple speech revisions. In addition, some thoughts are lengthy or cover substantial territory, as in the telling of a narrative, and may consequently require some internal organization.

The social setting also may raise the consequences of saying some-thing that is incorrect or socially inappropriate, as, for example, in school, making it more important to utter or not to utter specific con-tent. This, too, may make the cognitive job more difficult and result in added hesitation or revision, both of which add time beyond that "available" for the intended utterance.

There are no formal tests for assessing a person's communicative environment for its cognitive demand, but it is not difficult for clini-cians to evaluate this demand. Parents who converse with their chil-dren on abstract, confusing, or complex topics are usually easy to identify. The problem is that the children of such parents are usually also bright and academically inclined, and thus are likely to respond appropriately and with engagement. Nevertheless, the cognitive demands they are addressing may still interfere with their motor speech performance. In the absence of clearer tests of this variable, the mean length of parents' utterances and their mean word length will approximate the cognitive level of the child's environment.

In addition to the specific demands just mentioned, certain aspects of a person's home life may place such burdens on the person that vir-tually all areas of demand may be affected adversely. Violence in the home, alcoholism or other addictions, marital discord, or extreme poverty can all make a child's life unbearably difficult and can be expected not only to affect the child's fluency level but also to have a negative impact on the prognosis for treatment. Such a background will complicate in unpredictable ways the patterns of reaction and coping when the child becomes an adult.

As children grow into adults, these demands, which are original-ly part of the communicative milieu, become internalized. Although less influenced by the speech and reactions of those around him or her than as a child, the adult is more apt to struggle in speaking because of these internal values, feelings, perceptions, and thoughts. Evaluation of the adult who stutters with regard to environmental demands is consequently an exploration of his or her internal environment, a discussion of those inner experiences that elicit stuttering or exacerbate it, and a reevaluation of those beliefs (values, feelings, perceptions, and thoughts) he or she holds about stuttering. From this conversation, the client can develop a heightened awareness of his or her own inner life and the way it influences stuttering behaviors. It is the first step in becoming more aware of stuttering and the beginning of recovery.

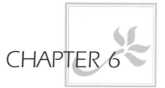

CHAPTER 6

Therapy for Children

The demands and capacities model (see Starkweather et al., 1990) provides a guide for the planning of therapy with young children. The goals are simple: increase the child's capacities in the motor, language, emotional, and cognitive areas, or let nature increase them through development, while at the same time reducing the demands of the child's communicative environment through counseling and training the child's parents, siblings, teachers, day care workers, and others who have an influence on the child.

The Preschool Child at Risk for Stuttering

Therapy for young preschool children is largely preventative—The goal is to prevent them from developing a chronic stuttering problem, whether they are at risk for or actually in the early stages of the disorder.

Planning Therapy

The first and most important element in preventing a child from developing a chronic stuttering problem is a thorough evaluation of the child's capacities and the demands that the child's environment is making on those capacities. With both quantitative and qualitative measures of demands and capacities, the clinician is ready to begin planning therapy.

It is important, however, to make sure that the techniques will be effective before committing both the parents' and the clinician's time and effort to a program of therapy. The existence of addictions or abuse present barriers to effective family therapy and should be either ruled out or dealt with before effective speech therapy can begin. Alcoholism and drug or other addictions in the family inhibit family members' capacities to be fully involved. Although each clinician will have an adopted policy with regard to these matters, in the long run we have found it to be more responsible to the client to refuse to work with the family until specific treatment is under way. The clinician will not be doing anything helpful by trying to brush these major sources of family tension and turmoil aside because it will be close to impossible to implement a prevention program. We believe it is naively optimistic to think that a child will benefit from a program of family therapy for a fluency problem while these more important issues remain unresolved. In many families, sexual and/or physical abuse are also problems that make it extremely difficult to accomplish any therapeutic goals. Children who are victims of these practices are being robbed of their childhood, and until they can begin to see some of that childhood coming back to them, it is unlikely that stuttering, which also robs the child of childhood, can be given the priority it deserves.

A useful strategy in ensuring that time will not be wasted is the "hypothesis-testing" approach. In this approach, the clinician decides first that specific changes in the child's capacities and in the environment's demands will be targeted. The clinician then chooses a particular strategy for achieving these changes. Before proceeding, the clinician tests the hypothesis that the chosen strategy will be effective in producing the desired change. For example, it may seem evident from the evaluation that a child's fluency will be increased if the parents could be taught to ask fewer questions requiring long, complex answers. To test the hypothesis that questions of this type are demanding for this child, the clinician can spend a half hour or so talking to the child, asking many of the kinds of questions that are suspected of stressing the child's fluency. The child's speech is recorded and measures are taken of his or her fluency level. Another session is planned in which the clinician asks none of the suspected questions. Again a recording is made and the child's fluency level is measured. If questions of this type are indeed demanding for this particular child, there should be a significant difference in the child's fluency level between the two sessions. A discovery of such a difference confirms the hypothesis. The clinician will then feel comfortable in asking the parents to make such a change because it is clear that it should improve the child's fluency. The evidence from such a positive finding makes a compelling argument that will help the clinician convince the parents, if they need convincing, that the chosen strategy is the one to follow.

If, on the other hand, there is little or no difference between the two sessions, the clinician should remain uncertain about the particular strategy. It is very important that the clinician not use an observation of little or no difference between the two test sessions to decide that the strategy will not work. It may yet work. There could be a number of reasons other than the hypothesis being tested why the two test sessions were not different. One obvious explanation for the negative result is that the clinician is not the parent and it is the parent who will be administering the strategy. This could be remedied by training the parent and having him or her administer the treatment. Of course, this begins to involve the parent in the kind of time and effort that the hypothesis testing is designed to avoid. Nevertheless, in the event of a negative result, a pair of test sessions with the parent seems like a reasonable next step. A second reason could be that the clinical setting is different from the home setting where the parent would be administering the strategy. The main point is not to think of the negative result as proving something. However, a series of negative results using different change agents in different settings does suggest that the strategy may not be effective.

The hypothesis-testing phase of intervention, which is poised between evaluation and management, need not last too long. Usually several sessions are sufficient to provide evidence that one or more strategies will be effective. If there is no such confirmation, then the clinician has to go forward with what seems like the best treatment, based on the evaluation.

Increasing Capacities

Children are growing rapidly during the preschool years, and all four of the areas of capacity will improve by themselves. Motorically, preschool children become more coordinated, and this means that they become better able to perform motor acts with a minimum of muscular effort. Linguistically, they are growing very rapidly in the early years, sometimes too rapidly for fluency, but their linguistic capacities for fluency—word finding, sentence formulation, and so forth—are also growing. Emotionally, they are learning to be less afraid of things and more comfortable in social situations. Cognitively, they are learning more about the world, about themselves, and about their place in the world. Not unimportantly, their sense of themselves in the family is also changing. Clinicians can capitalize on all this growth. Programs that seek only to modify the preschool child's environment so as to reduce demands can achieve remarkable success because the child's capacities are naturally growing at the same time.

In addition to allowing the child to mature, clinicians can do other things to help the process along and increase the child's capacities for fluency. The following section summarizes the role a good clinician plays in building up a child's capacities for fluency.

Increasing Motoric Skill

Building up the child's capacities for smooth and rapid speech movement seems like the most straightforward way to deal with stuttering. The coordination, speed of movement, and speech motor control that children need in order to speak fluently can be best practiced by having them speak fluently. Consequently, the clinician will give a child lots of opportunities to talk under circumstances where fluent speech is more likely to occur. In essence, this is the principle on which environmental manipulation is based—create or increase conditions that allow the child to talk fluently and encourage the child to talk in them. Although it might be tempting to try specific exercises, it is unlikely that any exercise will provide movements that are as close to the movements of speech as speech itself.

It is also important to take steps that will prevent the child from developing an attitude that speech is dangerous and something to be avoided, because such an attitude will tend to reduce the opportunities that the child has to practice under conditions that allow speech to be produced fluently.

Increasing Language-Performance Capacities

Children can be taught some of the language-performance skills that they need in order to speak more fluently. The two language skills that most often detract from fluency by occupying time are word retrieval and sentence formulation. Word retrieval can be developed by teaching children to use semantic categories and phonetic cues in the same manner as adults. For example, as a child searches for a noun, the clinician can suggest that he or she think about what can be done with the thing, how big it is, whether it is something that might be found in the home, what it is shaped like, and so forth. These semantic cues will eventually trigger the particular word. Another strategy is to prompt the child to think about the sound with which the word begins because often this phonetic cue helps in finding the word. With continued practice of this kind, the child's ability to find words should improve.

Sentence formulation can be quickened by making the rule-based grammatical structure of sentences more overt. For example, as a child struggles with a particular sentence, the clinician can remind the child what grammatical rule is being applied. With practice in making applying grammatical rules overtly, children can improve their grammatical formulation ability. Similarly, pragmatic skills can be increased by discussing the possibilities of how to say things differently in different situations.

Perhaps most valuable for the child who stutters is information about phonological rules and speech sound production. A working knowledge of speech production is very useful for the school-age child; for this reason the technique is described in detail in the next section on children in this group. The problem for the clinician dealing with a preschool child is how to make phonological knowledge simple enough so that the child can understand it. This can be done most easily by associating a fun-sounding and age-appropriate label with a type of speech sound. With this knowledge, children who stutter can gain some sense of empowerment over their speech mechanism. For example, sibilants are hissing sounds, plosives are popping sounds, and so on. See the discussion in the section titled "Moving Forward." In general, this technique is not appropriate for the young preschooler but may be useful for an older preschool child.

Increasing Emotional Capacities

Of all the capacities, the socioemotional area offers the most possibility for the preschool child. Parents who are well intentioned and engaged in helping their children usually understand them very well from an emotional point of view. Three types of emotional capacity—confidence, attitudes toward dysfluency, and sensitivity—can be worked on.

Building Confidence and Self-Esteem. In the preschool child, confidence and self-esteem seem related to the amount of attention the parents give to the child. Confidence is related to things the child does. The confident child expects to succeed at tasks. Self-esteem, on the other hand, is more a personal sense of worth.

Too much attention, or at least the tendency of over-attentive parents to do too much for their children, seems to undermine the child's sense of confidence. A child has to have opportunities both to fail and succeed in order to gain confidence. When the parent is "hovering" around the child, the child gets fewer opportunities to try things out, to experiment. Clinicians can be very helpful in this area in two ways. First, they can counsel the parents to ease off a little and let the child try new things. Parents should allow for mistakes and the lessons that come from them. Second, the clinician can provide opportunities for the child to be challenged at a level where he or she can succeed, particularly with regard to talking. It is, of course, the child's sense of confidence as a speaker that is most at risk when there is the possibility of a fluency problem.

Clinicians can also help build the child's confidence in speaking by appreciating aspects of the child's communication behavior that are not impaired. Complimenting children on the sweetness or power of their voice, on the enthusiasm with which they express ideas, on their choice of words, on their listening skills, or on their clarity of expression—none of which should be diminished by the presence of dysfluency—can help the children see that in many ways they are really *good* communicators. This can go a long way toward helping children not reach that dreadful conclusion that talking is just something they don't do very well. Fluency is not everything.

When parents pay too little attention to the child, the child's self-esteem diminishes. Consequently, it is not unusual to see a very confident child who has a low opinion of him- or herself. Many children who grow up in families where the parents are not available emotionally for one reason or another—alcoholism or addiction, preoccupation with their own problems, or difficulty in connecting to other people on an emotional level—can grow up to be highly competent individuals who know that they will succeed at most of the things they attempt, but they have a deep sense that they are not very worthwhile as people.

How much parental attention is too little? As with many important questions, the answer is "it depends." Some children seem to need a great deal of attention, whereas others seem not to need so much. One of the adjectives that the parents of children who stutter use to describe their child is "needy." Therefore, it sometimes is the speech clinician's rather difficult job to advise parents to find a level of attention that they can give to their child that is sufficient for the child but not exhausting for or likely to encourage resentment on the part of the parents. This can be a difficult balance.

One way would be to provide a brief period of high-quality attention on a regular basis. A child who is given 15 to 20 minutes each day of "special talking time," when they get completely focused parental attention, will come to look forward to it and derive much strength from it. In many ways, this is better than little snippets of attention throughout the day when the harried parent is actually trying to accomplish a number of other tasks. It is also easier on the parent to concentrate the attention in this way. If planned, it is less disruptive to the daily routine; because it is limited, it is usually something the parent can give to the child without becoming resentful and angry. In fact, many parents begin to look forward to this time. When this happens, the clinician has counseled well. We don't mean to suggest that the special talking time should be the only attention the child gets during a day. Young children need a lot of attention, but a special time that is set aside with no interruptions for phone calls, siblings, or chores is a wonderful gift for the child.

Developing Attitudes Toward Dysfluency. Young children develop the same values and attitudes as their parents. You can see it in the tendency a young child has to hold the same political and religious persuasions as his or her parents, even long before the child has been able to think with any sophistication about the actual issues. Other likes and dislikes—in food, music, art, friends, and activities—are all very easily picked up from the parents. It is only later, when the child gets into the rebellious teens, that independent values and attitudes will emerge. For the preschool child, attitudes arising during this part of the child's development seem to be adopted completely from parental attitudes.

In children who are at risk for developing stuttering, certain attitudes and beliefs can instigate a problem where there otherwise would be none or make a small problem much worse. The attitudes with which the adult or school-age child seem to have difficulty are as follows:

1. Dysfluent speech is the worst thing you can do;

2. People who are dysfluent aren't very smart/worthwhile/ attractive;

3. Stuttering is really a shameful thing to have; it means that you are bad in some way;

4. You should never mention stuttering to another person;

5. Stuttering is mysterious and frightening; and

6. Stuttering is a kind of personal weakness.

Although in preschool children these attitudes seem to be acquired from their parents, the older school-age child can acquire some of these same attitudes from the reactions of his or her peers.

A close look at the behavior of parents during the time when their child is stuttering, often best captured on videotape, can be very revealing. They may wince in pain, look away, abruptly leave the room, close their eyes, hold their breath, freeze in their conversational tracks, or look frightened. Sometimes these nonverbal reactions are quite subtle, but children at this age are very keenly tuned in to nonverbal behavior, and they pick up remarkably subtle nuances.

It is tempting for clinicians to try to modify these nonverbal behaviors directly, but, in the senior author's experience, this only makes matters worse. A parent who habitually looks away when the child stutters may, in trying not to look away, stare fixedly at the child. A parent who winces in psychological pain may adopt a look of forced relaxation. A parent who stops breathing when the child stutters may learn to breathe slowly and steadily but not naturally. The problem is that nonverbal behaviors are performed without thought, accompanying speech as a kind of dance to the tune of the language. Any attempt to make voluntary actions conscious produces a stilted version often overlaid with guilt.

It is better to talk at length to the parents about how they *feel* when the child stutters. As they describe their feelings to the clinician, they relive some of those feelings. The clinician listens attentively, actively, and with acceptance. How a person feels is how they feel, and it is understandable and common for parents to feel afraid, pained, ashamed, or impatient when the child speaks dysfluently. A support group for parents is even more effective in helping them realize that their feelings are common. Once it has developed some internal social structure and coherence, the group also supports its members by acknowledging that such feelings are acceptable. If they are allowed to feel in these ways, the parents will eventually work through these feelings, which actually are aspects of the grief cycle, until they accept that what their child is doing at that particular moment is speaking dysfluently or stuttering. They will then be ready to work on changing their behavior.

To counter the tendency for the child to develop an attitude that stuttering and dysfluency are awful and shameful signs of weakness or character defects, parents can be asked to model dysfluent speech when they talk to the child. They don't have to do this very often (once or twice a day is sufficient), just enough so that the child learns that speech can be dysfluent and that it isn't a shameful thing to do. It is best if the parents can model dysfluencies that are normal for the child's age rather than dysfluencies that are normal for an adult. For example, adults say "um," whereas children between ages 2 and 4 usually repeat whole words; therefore, the parents should repeat whole words. This may make the parents uncomfortable, however, and it is very important that they do not model discomfort in association with dysfluency. Consequently, the clinician should practice with the parents until it seems quite clear that the parents can repeat whole words without any accompanying sign of discomfort.

A well-known pattern in families where there is stuttering is the conspiracy of silence. This is the tendency for families not to mention the child's stuttering. In the past, some families were even advised by physicians and, sadly, by some speech pathologists not to mention it. The parents or the person advising them were afraid that bringing the stuttering out in the open would increase the child's discomfort. Actually, exactly the opposite happens. Children who grow up with a stuttering problem in a family where the problem is not mentioned come to believe that it is an unspeakable thing. This categorizes stuttering with topics such as bathroom behavior or sex, which are genuinely private matters. Stuttering does not belong in such a category; it is a distinctly public act. The dissonance between what the child hears him- or herself doing and the silence about it in the family is substantial.

In addition to learning that stuttering is somehow unmentionable, some of these children seem to conclude that it is inaudible. Most speech clinicians have seen adults who stutter who do not realize that their listeners can see and hear everything that they do when they stutter. There are two possible explanations for this. One is the well-known fact that people do not hear normal dysfluencies; these dysfluencies are not heard because they do not convey any information. Perhaps people who stutter hear their own stuttering behaviors in this way, rather than as the abnormalities that listeners hear. The other possibility is that children whose parents ignore their child's stuttering may inadvertently be teaching the child that the stuttering behaviors cannot be heard.

Desensitization. Clinicians can also reduce the impact that fear can have on fluency by desensitizing the child. There are two types of desensitization. The first type has as its goal a calming of fears, a reduction of shame, or a cooling of anger that may be interfering with fluency. By modeling discontinuous speech of a type that would be normal for the child's age, clinicians and parents show the child that this is not something to be afraid or ashamed of. By listening to the child express anger, clinicians and parents alike can allow the child to "have" the feelings and work through them.

The second type of desensitization is "toughening" the child to the environmental events that tend to be demanding of fluency. Usually introduced during the latter parts of therapy, this type involves increased audience size, interruptions from listeners, more open-ended questions, and a faster rate of speech from significant others. This enables the child to maintain fluency skills in the face of an increasingly demanding environment.

A very useful way to help children learn concepts or deal with issues that might be difficult is the group storytelling session. There is something very special about telling a story to a group of children. If the story is well written and is told with some dramatic flair, children are completely enthralled. During the storytelling, they seem to enter a different psychological state where they can experience vicariously some of the feelings expressed in the story. Feelings that would completely overwhelm the children in real life can be experienced without harm through this medium. It is quite useful to write a story with the purpose in mind of helping one particular child work through an issue in his or her life, and then tell the story to a group of children that includes the child with the problem. Appendix B contains a story written by a graduate student for telling to a group of children at risk for stuttering.

Increasing Cognitive Capacity

Three concepts can be helpful for the preschool child dealing with a fluency problem. The first is the idea of going slowly. The 2- or 3-year-old child who stutters is probably not very good at doing things slowly. It may be that the child actually doesn't have a good sense of doing things slowly; most children at this age do everything as fast as they can, perhaps because they can't do very many things as quickly as adults or older siblings. They have to keep trying to go as fast as possible, and the idea that some things, like talking, may actually be better accomplished by doing them more slowly will be unfamiliar to them.

Clinicians can introduce the child to this concept through arts-and-crafts activities, where many goals can be more easily reached through slower movement, or through stories. "The Tortoise and the Hare" is a story designed, it seems, for preschool children dealing with a fluency problem.

The second concept is quite similar—that some things happen better when you don't try so hard. This idea is a little harder to grasp than the idea of moving more slowly, and it is probably best to teach the slowing idea first, after which the idea of doing something gently comes a little easier. A pet such as a cat or hamster can often be used to teach these children about gentleness because the animals will squirm to get away if they are handled too roughly. After a brief session petting a small, soft animal, the clinician will find that it is much easier to teach a young child that he or she should touch, not press, with their tongue or lips in making a speech sound.

The third concept is that of taking turns. An aspect of sharing (sharing time), turn taking is also a concept or idea that the younger preschool child may not yet have learned. Because it is taking turns with speaking that is of concern here, the idea of using a talking stick[1] is very useful. The talking stick is introduced with some ceremony so that the children understand that it grants a certain power to the person who holds it. Then the clinician introduces a topic, such as the main idea in the story the children just heard. The child who has the

---

[1]The talking stick is used in Native American councils to grant the right to speak to whoever is holding the talking stick. When the stick is decorated in a way that signifies its spiritual importance, and when it has been introduced to the children with appropriate dignity, it can be a helpful reminder of whose turn it is.

stick is allowed to talk. Others must wait until the stick comes to them. The stick can be passed around the circle, or it can be given to each child by the leader. Children at this age find any idea easier to grasp if it is made more concrete in some way, and the talking stick, or any object that they can hold in their hands, helps to make it clear to them when it is their turn to talk or when they should wait. A toy microphone could also be used.

All these improvements in capacities for fluency will be helpful to the child in dealing with a demanding communication environment. In general, however, more progress is made by modifying the child's environment than can be achieved by teaching skills to him or her. There is a reason for this: These children are very young and skills of this sort are not particularly interesting to them. That doesn't mean they cannot learn, but rather that the clinician needs to figure out how to present the ideas and teach the skills in a way that is motivating.

Reducing Demands

Reducing demands is the first line of defense with young dysfluent children. It is the quickest, simplest, and least costly (in terms of both time and money) method for preventing a preschool child at risk for stuttering from developing the disorder. In addition, it is far more effective than adult therapy, both in the quantity and quality of outcome. Of all the adults who work long and hard to overcome their stuttering in most of the current fluency-shaping programs, only half or fewer succeed in the long term, and the quality of their success is low. They often talk in a slow, droning voice and have to monitor their speech movements constantly. This is not true for the preschool child who has completed a stuttering-prevention program. Most clinicians report close to 100% success in enabling the child to talk in a completely natural (not just natural-sounding) way, to talk spontaneously, without monitoring speech movements or "targets," and to talk at a normal rate and with a normal speech melody. In addition, very little relapse is reported for this population.

There are two reasons why decreasing environmental demands is so successful with the preschool child. First, they are still within the period of developmental plasticity. What they learn at 2, 3, or 4 years of age will change the way they talk permanently and without conscious control. This quality of change is also possible in the younger school-age child (e.g., a first grader), but by the second grade it is already difficult to achieve lasting change. This is discussed further in the section on the school-age child.

Second, the preschool child's environment is easy to control. These children live at home with their parents or, in some cases, with another family member, so most of the talking they do is to people who are deeply invested in their well-being and who are willing, indeed usually extremely eager, to do what they can. It is not usually difficult to get the parents to comply with the clinician's requests to modify the child's listening environment.

The Motor System

The most ubiquitous and powerful demand on the motor system is time pressure. The reasons for this have been spelled out already. Fortunately, there are a number of ways to reduce time pressure in a child's communicative environment. The most direct way is to teach the parents how to talk more slowly but in a natural way. The effects of slowed parental speech rate on fluency have been well documented (Stephenson-Opsal & Bernstein-Ratner, 1988). Although it is not clear why, the child's fluency improves when the parents are taught to talk more slowly. It could be simply that the slower parental rate creates an atmosphere where time pressure is reduced, thus lessening the parents' and the child's sense of urgency to communicate. It may also be that the child doesn't try to talk so fast when the parental model is slower. It is difficult to be certain because, as the child whose speech is full of dysfluency slows down, the dysfluencies decline and a more rapid rate of speech then occurs. In other words, it may look as though the child is actually talking faster because the speech is more continuous, although in fact it may be that the movements of speech are being made in a more leisurely way that reduces muscle activity levels.

When teaching parents to talk more slowly, clinicians in some cases will try to remove a number of odd by-products from the parents' speech before implementing the strategy. The first of these by-products is language effects. People talking more slowly seem to use language that is somewhat different from their usual style: They are likely to use shorter sentences and perhaps, along with the shorter sentences, a simpler syntactic structure. There is no need to correct this by-product. Although simpler language usually doesn't have much of an effect on children's fluency levels, in some cases it may improve fluency. It does sound quite natural to talk in this simpler way when talking slowly, and it can't hurt. Another by-product of slowed speech is a reduction in melodic variation, which can sound very stilted and boring. Parents should be trained to retain the normal rhythm and melody of their speech even when they are talking more slowly. Parents who cannot learn to slow down without introducing this robotic-sounding speech pattern probably should not use slowed rate as a fluency-enhancing strategy. When they do, the child usually notices and complains about it. It does sound pretty awful. When rhythm and melody are continued at normal levels, slowed speech doesn't sound bad at all; in fact, many report that it has an elegant quality. A third by-product of slowed rate is a "reading" style. The speaker, even though speaking spontaneously, sounds as though they are reading from a printed text. They say "eh" instead of "uh" for the indefinite article and "thee" for "thuh" for the definite article, even in front of consonants. There are other similar changes. It is best to remove these by-products before allowing parents to use slowed rate in front of their children.

Many parents try to slow down by inserting more frequent and/or longer pauses in their speech. When the velocity of speech movements is still fast, these inserted pauses create a machine-gun quality to speech that does not seem to have the same fluency-enhancing properties as speech that is genuinely "in slow motion" through a reduction in the velocity of movements. It is this slowed movement that is effective in producing an atmosphere of relaxation and reduced time pressure.

Many parents want to know how slowly they should talk. They also want to know how to tell when they are talking slowly enough. There is no specific rate. Because the object is to reduce time pressure on the child, one rule of thumb is to talk as slowly as the child talks. The clinician will know that the speech is not tending to speed the child up through convergence. The other rule of thumb is for the parent to talk slowly enough so that he or she feels a relaxation effect, which is quite noticeable because the speaker suddenly feels profoundly relaxed. Many parents who discover this find that it is a wonderful way to slow down and relax at any time. If the parent's speech urgency has been removed, this relaxation effect will occur and the time pressure on the child will be reduced.

Another source of time pressure is the rushed household. Apparently a ubiquitous feature of the modern family, the rushed household puts everything under time pressure, and the child's speech enters into this madness. It is remarkably easy to reduce time pressure from this source. Every family is different, of course, but in most families more time can be found so that the chores of the day still get done without the sense of rushing that seems to play such havoc with the speech of a child who has fluency problems. One family believed that most of their rushing was in the morning as they got the children dressed and ready for the day. We suggested that they get up 15 minutes earlier, which they reported as having remarkably good effects both on the child's fluency level and on their family life in general. Sometimes the best solution is a simple one. Other families will need to manage their time more efficiently. Most speech clinicians need only recall their time in graduate school to remember the tools that are necessary for good time management.

Another common source of time pressure is competition for speaking time among two or more children. Clinicians can help by teaching better turn-taking skills to the child, and parents are usually eager to have their children learn to stop interrupting.

Children who live in families where there is a lot of talking and where a high value is placed on verbal activity will usually be advanced in their language development. These "language overstimulation" cases (described in Chapter 4) use longer sentences and bigger words than their age peers. A reduction in the level of linguistic complexity in the child's speech will probably help in getting the child to slow down because the shorter sentences tend to be spoken more slowly. In general, however, it is not easy to get children to use a simpler grammar once they know the more complex one and have discovered its utility in expressing their ideas about the world around them. See the discussion below on reducing demands on the language system.

The Language System

Children whose language development is being overstimulated can be helped to become more fluent by a reduction in the amount of language they hear. Language, however, is the mediator of social interaction, and clinicians do not want to find themselves in the position of suggesting that parents communicate less with their children or become aloof from them. Consequently, it is useful to ask the parents to look for ways in which they and the child can have interactions that are mutually satisfying with less talking, for example, doing things that require less talking. The shared activity is a kind of interaction that leaves both parties feeling as if they have spent time with the other. Naturally, the goal is not to have the parent sit in stony silence. Talking is to be expected. The goal is to reduce the amount of talking without reducing the amount of time and interaction between parent and child.

The Socioemotional System

There are two broad categories of demands on the emotional system in preschool children—anxiety and excitement. Both are equally powerful. Neither can be entirely removed from the child's environment, nor is it necessary to do so, but a reduction, even in some cases a rather small reduction in either one of these two sources of arousal, can be helpful for a child at risk for developing a stuttering problem.

The sources of anxiety for a preschool child are somewhat different from those for an adult. The following events tend to make preschool children anxious: a move to a new house; a new baby-sitter, playschool, or day-care placement; illness or death in the family; fighting between parents; and the birth of a sibling. In most cases, these events cannot be prevented from occurring, although sometimes they can be postponed until after a child's speech has become fluent. In any case, the child can be prepared for these events by talking about them beforehand in a calm way and making sure that any questions or doubts are addressed. In the case of events that cannot be anticipated, parents can alleviate a great deal of children's anxiety by giving them lots of attention, reassuring them about doubts they may have, and generally being supportive. The problem is that these events are usually upsetting to parents also; this is where the speech clinician can be quite helpful. By talking to the parents about these events, whether they are anticipated or not, the clinician can help the parents deal with the events in a genuinely calmer way, which will have a beneficial effect on the child's speech.

There are also a number of sources of excitement—vacations, birthday parties, visits to or by grandparents, a parent arriving home from a trip or even from work. All of these events can raise the child's level of excitement to a point where the fluency threshold is exceeded. Clinicians do not want to make a child's life bland and do not advise parents to remove excitement from the child's life. On the other hand, parents often try to "hype up" situations in advance in order to make them more fun for the child. Clinicians should advise parents not to do this. They can continue to do most of the things they want to do with their child, but they can present them, plan for them, and discuss them afterward in a calmer tone so the child has just as much fun but doesn't get so wildly excited before the event. In some cases certain events can be postponed until the child is no longer dysfluent or they can be modified so as to make them a little less stimulating (e.g., having a smaller birthday party).

The Cognitive System

Questions that require long, complex answers, recalling a sequence of events, or selecting one event to discuss from a number of events all place demands on the child for thought that may well interfere with his or her linguistic or motor performance. "Tell Mommy what you did at school today" requires selection, sequencing, and narration. "Tell Daddy what you told me about the little girl at playschool" involves recall, selection, and repetition of a story without being boring or losing detail. These kinds of questions tend to provoke dysfluency, and parents are well advised to try to reduce their frequency. Parents instead can provide opportunities for the child to speak on a particular topic, perhaps indirectly by saying something to the child of the same kind and then waiting. If the child doesn't feel like talking, he or she should be allowed the opportunity to remain silent. This will increase the spontaneity of utterance and thus promote fluency. Usually the story will come out, although it may take a little more time. Once parents discover that they can learn everything they want to know about their child's day without specifically requesting it, both the parents' lives and the child's life are improved.

Demand speech is an old concept that has recently been augmented. In some of the older texts, demand speech referred to asking the child to say a particular thing, such as telling a story or reciting a poem or set piece. These types of speech acts are difficult for a child with a stuttering problem to perform and are best reduced to infrequent occurrences. There are other types of demand speech, such as "say thank you" or "say goodbye," that put words in the child's mouth, taking from them the responsibility for their own speech. Translating for bilingual parents, or any form of speaking for someone else, is a type of demand speech. Where circumstances in the child's family are such that the child is often asked to talk in a nonspontaneous way, it will be difficult for the child to be fluent. Parents should find better ways to accomplish their goals than by using demand speech. Modeling politeness works just as well as requesting it. Usually the other forms of demand speech can be dropped altogether.

Criteria for Discharging the Preschool Child

Two criteria need to be satisfied in order to discharge a preschool child at risk for stuttering: Speech should be completely normal over a period of at least 6 weeks,[2] and the parents need to feel confident that there is no longer any reason to be concerned about the child's stuttering. In some cases, the child's speech can contain some residual stuttering behavior, but if progress has been good and the parents show evidence of being particularly well equipped to handle whatever remains, a change to monitoring rather than intervention seems appropriate. Parents need to be advised that there will be times when there may be a surge of normally dysfluent speech; if they have been trained in the differences between normal and abnormal dysfluency, this should not seem threatening to them. These surges of normal dysfluencies often follow spurts of language development where increased sentence and word lengths place demands on the child's ability to make the rapid and smooth movements that fluent speech requires.

Clinicians also should advise parents to call whenever anything changes in the child's speech behavior or if some particularly stressful situation is anticipated. A little telephone counseling can go a long way toward helping the parent deal with these situations so as to avoid an increase in the child's dysfluency.

The School-Age Child

School-age children whose stuttering has become chronic are a particularly difficult group to treat. Too old for most of the prevention strategies and too young for the self-confrontation involved in adult therapy, they require creative strategies if they are not to fall between the cracks. The difficulty stems from the kind of attitude toward

---

2For older preschool children (ages 4½ to 6), this period should be extended to 3 to 4 months.

dysfluency that they are likely to have at this age. These children are "chasing after the fluency god" (Reed, n.d.) They would rather do anything than display their stuttering behavior. As a result, they are delighted when they come upon a new "trick" that enables them to talk without stuttering. They may tell the clinician, as one child did, that they have found the cure for "it." They are so happy at having discovered that they can say a word without stuttering on it if they perform some rhythmic movement at the same time, or change a word, or look away, or click their tongue, that the reinforcement for these learned behaviors is very powerful. In addition, this "learning process" is often avoidance conditioning (see Starkweather, 1996), which is particularly difficult to extinguish. As a result, clinicians need to use powerful techniques to help these children learn to talk in an easy way.

Management

There are a number of techniques for helping the school-age child who stutters develop a healthier set of attitudes about stuttering, speech, and social life in general. In addition, there are specific techniques that will help such a child learn to speak more easily. Both are important, but the work on attitudes is by far the most important part of treatment for this age group. Many clinicians who work only on the child's dysfluent behavior spend years trying to achieve change with little or no success. These children's belief that being fluent is more important than anything else will lead them to perform many behaviors that are much more abnormal than stuttering.

At the same time, because the child can see nothing but the need to be fluent, it is often necessary for motivational purposes to begin by teaching the child some ways to talk more easily. The clinician needs to lighten the child's burden a little to demonstrate competence. Children at this age are not impressed by credentials; they want results, and fast! The clinician needs to choose strategies that promote easier talking without buying into the child's misperception that fluency is more important than anything else.

There are many different ways to approach the school-age child, so the methods suggested here should not be taken to be the only way. They are simply techniques that have been found to be effective in one way or another.

It can be useful to begin by making the child aware of two aspects of his or her stuttering—the time stuttering behaviors take up and the kind of abnormality the behaviors display to listeners. This should be done fairly. If the child has some behavior that does not take up too much time and does not display abnormality, the clinician needs to acknowledge this. These more subtle behaviors can be treated when the child has become more fluent and is more receptive to the idea that they cost too much in effort. The child first has to experience the relief of giving up struggle behaviors, and it will be easier for the clinician to succeed in this on the basis of the time they take up or of how abnormal they look.

Moving Forward and Repairing

"Repair" techniques involve modifying the stuttering behavior at the moment that it is happening by substituting normal speech-production behaviors for stuttering behaviors. Sometimes the movements are correct but are made with excessive muscle tension; in this case, the repair consists of reducing muscular tension, often by slowing momentarily and letting the word out rather than pushing it. Struggling to talk is abnormal, so a reduction of struggle and a more "passive" role in talking is appropriate. The child is already doing too much and needs to learn how to do less.

There are different repair techniques for different types of stuttering and for different types of sounds. For example, a laryngeal block, which could prevent forward movement on any voiced sound, can be modified by teaching the child to gradually reduce the pressure behind the vocal folds until it dips below the Valsalva threshold. At this point, the vocal folds will begin vibrating and the word will seem to just come out by itself. The child needs to learn to let this happen.

Similar techniques designed to reduce muscle activity level and pressure can be used to repair other stuttering behaviors at the moment they are occurring, that is, without backing up and saying the word over again.

Most sounds involve two or three elements. Vowels, for example, require that the mouth be in a certain position and that the voice be activated. Semivowels (/r, l, y, w/) involve those two elements, but there also is a movement away from the initial position to the position associated with the next vowel. For fricative sounds (/f, v, th, s, z, sh, zh/) there is a particular position, airflow, and then, for the voiced fricative, the additional activation of voice. For plosives (/p, t, k, b, d, g/) and affricates (/tsh, dzh/) there is again a specific position and airflow, with or without voice, followed by a rapid movement to the next sound. The /h/ sound is quite unique in its manner of production. First the position for the following vowel is taken, then airflow is begun, and then voicing, which seems out of order. Using these simplified labels and extremely simple descriptions of features can help the child organize the process of speech sound production so that he or she will spend speech time making the movements of talking rather than the movements of stuttering.

Children of school age find it helpful to learn about the various speech sound categories. There is a genuine sense of power that they have by knowing that the sound they are trying to say is an affricate or a semivowel. Once they have learned how each of the sound categories are made, they can contrast the movements of forward-moving speech with the movements of stuttering. With practice, they can learn to substitute the forward-moving movements for the stuttering behaviors.

When the knowledge of phonological skill is coupled with a "moving-forward" strategy, the child will find that he or she wastes much less time on extraneous behavior. Moving forward means making the movements needed to produce the features of a specific speech sound and then, once it has been produced, moving on to the next speech sound. Both adults and children can save large amounts of time that previously had been spent on extraneous behaviors such as backing up or taking a deep breath by learning to simply move forward in their speech. Sometimes there is a tendency for more stuttering to appear at first because some of the child's extraneous behavior may have been learned as a way of hiding the stuttering behavior. The child will have to learn to take a little risk of stuttering, to learn that it is OK to stutter a little as progress is made toward fewer extra behaviors. This will also be a beginning for changing attitudes away from the "fluency is everything" belief.

This approach depends to a certain extent on the child being somewhat mature. He or she has to take the responsibility for doing what has to be done at the level of movement. For some, particularly the younger school-age child, this may be difficult. In addition, as a defense against the pain of stuttering, some children abdicate whatever responsibility they may have had. They conclude that there is nothing they can do about it and trying to do something about it seems always to fail, so they won't try any more. For children with this less mature attitude, whether it has been learned as a strategy or not, an approach using systematic rewards may be useful.

Normalizing Dysfluencies (Dysfluency Shaping)

A different approach to relief from the burden of stuttering is more appropriate for the younger or less mature child (perhaps the first or second grader) who may not be able to understand or appreciate the efficiency and increased normality of the moving forward and repairing strategy just described.

In this approach, the clinician identifies a particular feature—usually the most abnormal one or the one that takes up the most speech time—of the child's stuttering behavior and targets it for removal. The clinician then systematically rewards the child every time he or she stutters without using this particular feature. If an appropriate reinforcer is used, that is, a tangible item that the child wants (the senior author advocates dimes), the child will start to be more aware of what he or she is doing and will begin using the particular device or behavior less and less. When it is no longer being used, the child's speech is a little bit closer to being normal. A second behavior then will be targeted for removal, and again stuttering that does not contain this behavior is reinforced systematically until the targeted abnormality is gone. The clinician continues to do this until the dysfluent behavior is normal in character.

Controlling Fluency

With older children or children who have not responded well to the less "invasive" techniques described above, fluency-control techniques may be appropriate. Three types—rate control, easy onset, and blending—appear to be useful. Rate control can be taught in three stages. The first stage (*slow rates*) is learning how to talk more slowly. As with the training of parents in speaking slower, the child learns to talk more slowly not by inserting pauses, which break up the natural rhythm of speech, but by slowing the movements of speech, which will reduce general muscle tension. All children are familiar with slow motion and super-slow motion from the movies. Clinicians can model how speech sounds when it is performed in super-slow motion, and children find little difficulty in imitating this way of talking. After the child has learned how to talk in super-slow motion, speech can be speeded up to slow motion. It is not a good idea to have the child use slow-motion speech when actually talking to people. It should be learned and practiced in the clinic as a first step but not be used as a way to talk with people.

The second stage (*rate control*) is gaining increased control over speech rate. The child practices talking at super-slow motion, slow motion, and normal speed. It doesn't take children very long to learn how to do all three rates when asked.

The third stage (*cued rate control*) is to teach the child to slow down—either to slow motion or to super-slow motion—when he or she needs to (i.e., when he or she feels that it is going to be difficult to talk) and then to speed up again as soon as he or she is past that point. With practice, children get very good at this and can slow down for a half second to get through a particular sound at the beginning of the word and then be back to a normal speech rate before the word is finished. Listeners will hardly be aware that the child is slowing, a fact that the child should verify by interviewing several listeners.

These techniques of rate control can be taught even to very young children, usually through metaphor. In those circumstances where the child's parents are unavailable to carry out a program of environmental modification in the home, because of language difficulties or cultural differences, preschool children can be taught this and other direct fluency-control techniques.

Clinicians can also help school-age children understand the concept of slowing down at certain times by comparing it to driving in heavy traffic. Not just slowing down, but the ability to control the rate at which the child is talking and to vary the rate for the circumstances (cued rate control) are useful techniques for the older school-age child.

Working on Attitudes

For children who have begun to think of themselves as poor speakers or as having no control over their speech, some cognitive retraining is useful. At this age, when peer evaluation becomes very important, the child who gets no attention or negative attention from peers is likely to feel bad about him- or herself. Speech clinicians have a number of ways of dealing with this situation, but all begin with listening.

People are validated by listening. During a conversation, the partners present their ideas, a piece of themselves. When a person's ideas are truly heard he or she feels connected to the listener. This is just as true for school-age children as it is for adults. As a result, through good listening the parent, clinician, teacher, or friend has an opportunity to make the child who stutters feel validated as a person. This also presents a wonderful opportunity to structure the listening in such a way that the child feels validated not only as a person, but as a speaker as well. It is this structured listening that is meant by the term listening therapy. It is worth noting that listening therapy, although originally devised for the practicing clinician, can easily be applied by any conscientious and concerned listener. There are four stages in listening therapy.

Stage 1 is listening to the person. In this stage, all the listener has to do is listen to the person, which means actively listening, paying attention to what the person is saying, and being genuinely interested. Pretending to be interested doesn't work very well. This stage sometimes can be difficult. One 8-year-old wanted to talk only about professional wrestling, which he found extremely interesting. It was quite a stretch for his clinician to learn the names of some of the professional wrestlers and watch a few wrestling matches on TV in order to develop enough of an interest in the subject so that the child would feel that the clinician genuinely was listening, but it paid off. This child's self-esteem developed rapidly from a state nearing clinical depression to where he was taking an active interest in schoolwork again for the first time in many months. Eventually, too, his interests widened, the passion over wrestling was left behind, and the clinician could return to watching episodes of "Nova" on PBS.

Stage 2 involves listening to the speech. As soon as the child's sense of self-esteem starts to lift a little—often evidenced by how willing the child is to talk—the listener can shift from showing his or her appreciation for what the child is saying to showing appreciation for aspects of the child's communicative behavior. This may be the quality of the voice, the enthusiasm with which he or she expresses ideas, the clarity of articulation, or the choice of words. Whatever is normal about a child's communicative behavior can be applauded. The goal is to help the child develop a better perspective as a speaker. Speech production, or sounds, may not be fluent, but many other aspects of communication are fine. Through the clinician's appreciation of these aspects, the child will learn that he or she isn't such a bad talker after all; the problem lies with one part of speech.

Stage 3 is listening to the stuttering. Once it is evident that the child's belief that he or she is a poor speaker has lessened, the listener can start focusing more on the child's stuttering pattern. It will become evident immediately that not all stuttering is equally abnormal, time consuming, or effortful. Some stuttering is better than other kinds. The listener can then begin to show appreciation for the ways in which the child stutters that are better than others by saying things such as "I really like the way you stuttered on that; it sounded nice and easy (or slow, or comfortable)."

Stage 4 is self-listening. The listener begins to shift the child's awareness toward self-listening and, at the same time, to incorporate the values expressed in Stages 2 and 3. The child will learn to listen to his or her own speech and to hear all the things that are normal or excellent about it. The same is true of stuttering behavior. The child can learn to hear stuttering that is easier or more normal sounding or briefer and to appreciate the fact that at a particular moment his or her stuttering behavior was better than usual.

When the four stages of listening therapy are finished and the child's sense of self-esteem and confidence as a speaker has lifted, the clinician might want to introduce or return to the moving forward and repair strategy described earlier. A child will find it much easier to make changes in his or her speech if the negative attitudes and beliefs have been removed or at least softened.

Dealing with Teasing

For very young preschool children, teasing is not so serious. They tease each other about minor foibles and differences such as having bright red hair. It is not such a bad thing for stuttering to be categorized in this way. This usually remains true during the earliest school years as well. By the time the child is 8, and through the fifth and sometimes sixth grades, teasing can be a major problem. The opinions of peers are now very important, and when those opinions are negative and expressed directly through teasing, the effect on the child can be devastating. Teasing can lead to severe depression, and it is at this age that some psychological referrals may be useful to help the child cope with the many social difficulties that stuttering presents.

There are several approaches to this problem. Probably the most effective way to deal with teasing is by obtaining help from the child's teacher. Teachers are usually quite willing to teach a lesson about respect for others to the whole class. These lessons are usually effective in removing teasing behavior for nearly all of the students. Sometimes, of course, there is an insecure child who bolsters his or her fragile ego by bullying others. These individuals will respect authority, because that is what they wish to have, and will respond to traditional discipline, although it may have to be repeated.

Another useful strategy for dealing with teasing is to remind the child of the various options that are available. The child being teased can tell the authorities (usually the teacher), talk to their parents, or tell the teaser very seriously that he or she doesn't like to be treated that way. The senior author asks his clients to supply various alternatives and then choose one. The response that will work best depends on the situation and on the person being teased. It is helpful for the child to realize that there are many choices, because they often feel trapped in the situation. Most children feel good about themselves when they decide not to hit the teaser (the clinician can provide a little advice in this case, too). The child whose stuttering is mild may be able to deal with teasing in the best way, by talking (teasing back, telling how he or she feels, etc.), but the child whose stuttering is severe may not choose talking as a way of dealing with the problem. The child who is strong may be able to intimidate the teaser, whereas the child who is not so strong may want to choose another strategy. Clinicians, parents, and teachers can be an important source of support for the child being teased by listening to the child, acknowledging how much it hurts and how unfair it is, and steering the child away from selected solutions that will do more harm than good.

A Special Word to Parents

Although this book is written for several kinds of readers, including aspiring speech clinicians, we hope that the lay public will also find it useful in their quest to understand better either their own stuttering or that of friends or family. For that reason, we consider the role of parents in a more general way. There are many things that parents can do to help the child who is stuttering. First, if it hasn't been done already, the parent needs to find support and perhaps even training in talking to their child about stuttering. The child needs to feel that when he or she is having a problem with stuttering, a parent is someone to go to for support, not judgment and criticism. This is a vital consideration. The child who gets only criticism (verbal or nonverbal) from his or her parents will tend to feel ashamed of the stuttering, try to hide it from others, and consequently engage in a wide variety of coping behaviors that in the long run will only make the stuttering worse. On the other hand, the child who feels that he or she can approach the parent and be heard has an outlet for the load of bad feelings that stuttering can generate.

Parents can also fight some of the battles that the child may be too young to fight for him- or herself. Sometimes parents can be helpful in explaining to other significant adults, such as grandparents or siblings, that the child has a stuttering problem, is working on it, and needs support rather than criticism. At the same time, it is important for parents to stop fighting battles and to stop being the child's voice to the outside world when the child is old enough to do these things for him- or herself. As a speech clinician, the senior author often gets phone calls from people seeking an appointment who introduce themselves and say that their son or daughter stutters. After the appointment is made, the author will ask how old the child is and be startled to hear the mother say 32 or some similarly mature age. Protection of this kind only further undermines the self-confidence of a person who stutters.

The parents of preschool children are the major agents of change for their children. It is not a good idea, however, for parents of older children to remind them to "use your slower speech now," or "don't forget to repair your stuttering behaviors." It takes only a few occurrences before this kind of reminding becomes nagging and the child tunes it out. In the end this "help" doesn't do any good anyway, and it has chipped away at what the child really needs: support, encouragement, and acknowledgement that the parent realizes he or she is working hard at overcoming stuttering. Many of the resources for persons who stutter listed in Appendix C offer help and guidance for parents as well.

The desperation that many parents feel can lead them to try many nonproductive strategies to overcome it. Where there has been a past pattern of sharp criticism or even rejection by the parent over stuttering, he or she needs to see that the more positive route will be more helpful to the child in the long run.

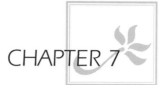

CHAPTER 7

Therapy for Adults

Nonavoidance Therapy

In the 1950s, Charles Van Riper began to formalize a method of treatment for stuttering that was based on his own personal experiences with the disorder. After a number of refinements, this method was consolidated and described in *The Treatment of Stuttering* (1973). In essence, it consisted of helping the person who stuttered confront his or her disorder, learn about it, and, with support and encouragement, learn how to develop an easier, less effortful way of stuttering. The outcome of these "stuttering modification" treatments (see Figure 7.1 on page 146) was difficult to quantify, but many were successful in teaching an easier way of stuttering. Typically there were tiny and almost unnoticeable residual behaviors that were not quite normal but were not a problem for the client. Speech was easier for these clients, and they were usually satisfied with the treatment. Some tendency to regress was present, but it was small, and the tools for dealing with it were provided as part of the treatment.

A major difficulty with Van Riper's stuttering modification approach was that it took a long time for clients to recover when they were treated in the typical weekly or biweekly session format. Some attempts to administer this type of therapy in an intensive format were made (Breitenfeld & Lorenz, 1995), and, although they tended to produce much more rapid change, the tendency toward regression seemed to be higher than with nonintensive programs (Prins, 1970).

Therapeutic Techniques Based on Control

In the 1960s and 1970s, Van Riper's influence began to wane as the influence of behaviorism took over the field. A number of behavioral treatments were developed (Brutten & Shoemaker, 1967; Shames & Florance, 1980), and a systematic speech modification program designed to shape the entire speaking behavior from highly discontinuous speech production to smooth and "stutter-free" speech was published by Webster (1972). The program was typically administered in an intensive residential setting. Many speech clinicians were trained in this procedure, and it has been very widely used. The results were considerably easier to quantify and suggested a very high rate of success in the short term but a strong tendency to regress to previous behavior in the long run. Modifications in the program, specifically the provision of "booster sessions," helped partially to alleviate the tendency to regress.

A number of therapy programs are currently available that teach the adult who stutters a new way of talking that does not include dysfluent behavior. The major forms of control therapies are "airflow therapy" (Schwartz, 1976), "stutter-free therapy" (Shames & Florance, 1980), and "precision fluency shaping" (Webster, 1972). Although they vary in the emphasis they place on different therapeutic elements, they share the same basic goal—teach the person a new way of talking so that they won't stutter at all. In precision fluency shaping, which is the best known of these control therapies, speech is systematically slowed down, and the person is taught to touch the articulators more lightly, to accentuate voicing by keeping the vocal folds in vibration for a greater percentage of speech time, and to breathe in a slower, calmer way. These techniques are partially effective. Typically, after several weeks of intense treatment, the person is able to talk in the new way, and the stuttering behavior is absent, at least temporarily (Webster, 1972).

However, there are several problems with these approaches. First, one has to concentrate very hard. The natural way of talking is to think about the thoughts that you are communicating and leave the process of speech production on automatic pilot. Speech evolved in just this way so that we could communicate efficiently. Second, and perhaps as a result, the relapse rate for these programs is very high, at least 30% for precision fluency-shaping (Webster, 1972),[1] and data regarding the other two have not been published in professional journals. Third, the

---

[1]Although the published reports indicate a 30% relapse rate, the personal experience of a number of clinicians suggests that it is considerably higher than this, at least 50%. In addition, the initial success rate is perhaps 65%. The difficulty is the matter of defining what is meant by success in the first place, and then defining and identifying those who have relapsed.

way in which the person talks after such therapy is typically slow, lacks melody and inflection, and often sounds stiff and stilted.

In a recent experiment, Franken, Peters, and Tettero (1989) compared the reactions of listeners to the speech of people who stuttered before and after treatment in one of these programs. Surprisingly, most listeners preferred to hear the stuttering behavior that preceded treatment rather than the new way of talking, which, although it was free of stuttering behaviors, lacked the spontaneity and melody of normal speech. Even more recently, Kalinowski, Noble, Armson, and Stuart (1994) compared naturalness ratings (see Martin, Haroldson, & Triden, 1984) before and after treatment in the precision fluency shaping program. Even though the clients' speech was free of stuttering, it was rated as less natural than before treatment.

Many clinicians are now trying to develop techniques for teaching speech that *sounds* natural as a final aspect of therapy. In some cases, a more natural-sounding speech pattern is attainable, although it still does not feel natural to the speaker (Franken, Konst, Boves, & Rietveld, 1995).

Integrated Approaches

In the 1980s and 1990s, most practicing clinicians integrated the speech modification and stuttering modification approaches (T. Peters & Guitar, 1991; Starkweather, 1994), and this seems to have led to improved naturalness and a reduction in the tendency to regress. The integrated approach was not only widely used, it was incorporated into a "best practices" paper (Starkweather, Blood, Peters, St. Louis, & Westbrook, 1993), which was eventually approved as a policy of the American Speech–Language–Hearing Association.[2] The integrated approach seems to yield a higher level of satisfaction on the part of clients, although little real outcome data are available to substantiate these conclusions. A survey of practicing clinicians indicated that nearly all of the respondents described themselves as using an "integrated" approach (Starkweather, 1994).

The integrated approaches teach clients the techniques of easy onset, slowed rate, and blending but also incorporate self-confrontation, attitude adjustment, and exploration of feelings. Clinicians who employ these therapies do not strive for speech that is completely free

---

[2]This paper is reproduced in its entirety in Appendix A of this book.

of dysfluency, arguing that normal speech is peppered with dysfluencies. The goal is speech that is comfortable for the client and as fluent as can be achieved without using methods that may be harmful in the long run. Some, but not constant, vigilance is required. The client is given considerably more choice about when and where to use the techniques that are taught. Most importantly, the nonavoidance techniques of pseudostuttering, self-confrontation and understanding, and reduction of fear and avoidance are combined with the fluency-enhancing techniques of slower speech rate, easier onset of utterance, and continuous voicing.

Integrated therapies also do away with some of the harmful practices of the more extreme control therapies. One example of such a method is the indoctrination that often characterizes the control therapies. This indoctrination is an attempt to make use of the well-known "placebo effects" on stuttering. Stuttering is remarkably susceptible to suggestion. When a person who stutters believes that he or she is being given the latest, most scientifically impeccable treatment, there is a strong tendency for the person's speech to improve This placebo effect has nothing to do with the therapy that is being administered, and it will wear off in time. Many practitioners of control therapies spend considerable effort to convince their clients that the treatment they are receiving is the only effective form. This hard sell does help in producing fluent speech, but the effect does not last. When the placebo effect wears off, the person is left with speech that is, at best, disappointingly worse than anticipated. In some cases, when the person was led to expect complete fluency, he or she is devastated by the poor final result. In addition, when a hard sell approach is used, there is a tendency for the client to feel that the failure was his or her fault. Responsible clinicians present their approaches to clients in a realistic manner. Clients may make slower progress, but the progress they do make is less likely to be lost. Some tendency to regress after treatment is to be expected, but a responsible clinician will explain this before therapy begins and help the client learn what the future may hold in a realistic description.

Transfer and Maintenance

Whatever modification therapy form is used, it is necessary to transfer the new way of talking and the new way of feeling about stuttering into real speech situations as they arise in everyday life. Most individuals who stutter have no difficulty in achieving fluent or nearly fluent speech in the clinic, regardless of the approach used. The difficulty is in getting this new way of talking and thinking about stuttering to be a part of the person's life. The problem of transfer is difficult in control therapies because of the need to concentrate on the process of speech production. This concentration becomes considerably more difficult when the client is confronted by one of his or her old difficult situations. As soon as he or she enters the speech situation, the client is flooded with a set of stimuli that elicit the old patterns of behavior. Usually, these situations also elicit fear because in the past they have often resulted in the person stuttering badly and feeling humiliated or ashamed. As the fear rises, the ability to concentrate on the behavioral targets of the control therapy is reduced and the person loses control. In other words, control techniques are most difficult to use when they are most needed.

One useful technique to help the person who stutters continue to learn how to speak better, and one that applies to all forms of therapy, is *the development of a problem-solving attitude* in the client. An individual who has been able to see the stuttering as his or her problem and one that he or she can solve begins to develop an attitude of personal responsibility that is most helpful. Upon finding her- or himself stuttering a little more, he or she takes some time to try to understand what he or she is doing, thinking, and feeling at the time. The client may then purposefully reenter the same situation to reexperience the feelings and behaviors and, in this way, work through the problem. A person in control therapy can also identify the situation that is giving him or her trouble and practice achieving behavioral targets in the situation until it is no longer a problem.

Another useful tool is the *designated listener*. In this technique, the person who stutters identifies one person to whom he or she talks on a daily basis. This person is the designated listener (DL). The person who stutters then talks to the DL, practicing whatever behavior or attitude client and clinician believe to be ready for transfer. The DL is usually not told that he or she has been assigned this role. As soon as the person who stutters has reached a specified level of achievement with the DL, another DL is selected, and the client practices with that person, in addition to the first DL. This goes on until a hierarchy of DLs is available and the person who stutters is talking in the new way to a wide range of individuals. At a certain point, everyone becomes a DL.

A third concept that has become useful in maintaining the gains made in therapy is the *dental model* (Blood, 1993). Stuttering is somewhat like tooth decay—something about which you always need to be alert. This idea means that people who stutter should be made aware that, no matter what the method, recovery from stuttering involves slipping back into old habits on some occasions. Consequently, it is useful after therapy is completed to schedule a person periodic checkups. When clients are told that this is the model they will be following when they begin therapy, it keeps the door open to people who are having trouble maintaining gains. One of the most difficult problems with stuttering is that people who have been through therapy and succeeded but who then slip back into old patterns feel ashamed to see the speech clinician again. They seem to see the failure of the treatment as a personal failure and do not contact the clinician. Others are simply angry that the treatment has not "worked" and dismiss it as worthless. In fact, with a prescheduled checkup and a relatively brief refresher all of the progress made in the therapy can often be regained. The dental model has proven quite useful in dealing with relapse.

Alternatives to Speech Therapy

Self-Help

Two additional developments have had a major impact on stuttering treatment and therapy. The first, as mentioned in Chapter 1, was the rise of the self-help movement, including groups targeted at helping people who stutter. Many people who stuttered, often displeased with the treatment they had received by well-meaning but uncertain clinicians, joined together in mutual support in groups such as The National Stuttering Project.[3] These organizations have been around for a number of years, but in the 1980s they began to grow in size and influence. Their value to people who stutter derives, in part, from the powerful feeling of support that people feel when they come together with others like themselves. There is no question that this feeling of acceptance allows people who stutter to feel freer than they do when talking to the general public and, as a result, their speech often im-

---

[3]A list of these resources is included in Appendix C.

proves dramatically.[4] Such a powerful therapeutic force cannot and should not be overlooked by clinicians interested in doing everything they can to help clients talk more easily and feel heard.

Few strategies are more effective in helping the adult who stutters learn how to stop denying and accept the reality of stuttering than to be faced with a roomful of people struggling and dealing with the same hurdles. Meeting together and talking with others about one's stuttering while feeling warmth and acceptance is both uplifting and instructive.

Personal Growth Movements

A second development of the 1980s, less widely known but gaining in influence in the general public, is the rise in importance of a variety of personal growth groups, including 12-step programs modeled on Alcoholics Anonymous. The success of these programs (and we have heard there are now over 100 different 12-step recovery programs) in helping individuals is remarkable (Beattie, 1990a).

A 12-step program for people who stutter—Compulsive Stutterers Anonymous—was described by Reed (n.d.) but is not widely known outside the Chicago area. Some of the elements of 12-step recovery programs may be difficult for speech clinicians and people who stutter to accept. These are programs of spiritual growth, and, although not religious in any formal sense, aspects of the program may seem so to some individuals. Nevertheless, the power of these programs in helping people recover from serious problems cannot be denied. From our own personal experience with these programs, it seemed worthwhile to incorporate elements of 12-step recovery into the treatment of stuttering. This approach is explored more fully later in this chapter under the section The Process of Recovery.

Devices That Reduce Stuttering

There are a number of devices on the market that people who stutter can wear that make it easier for them to talk. In most cases, the person

---

[4]It should be noted that for a few individuals the opposite occurs. As they feel freer to be themselves, they hide their stuttering less. The result is increased overt stuttering behavior.

wears a set of headphones and either a throat microphone or a microphone that is positioned in front of the mouth. These devices vary
somewhat in how they work and what they accomplish. Some merely
amplify the voice and feed this amplified signal to the hearing mechanism. Simple amplification like this has a moderate effect on some
individuals. Other devices alter the signal in some way before repre-
senting it to the speaker's ears. There are two types of these devices—
delayed auditory feedback (DAF) and frequency altered feedback
(FAF). The DAF devices delay the signal slightly before sending it
back to the speaker, which results in the sensation that the individual
is speaking in a place with an echo. Speaking with such a device slows
the person's speech by drawing out the vowel sounds and alters the
quality of speech in a few other ways. For listeners, the effect is a kind
of droning quality.

In the FAF devices, the signal is altered in its frequency so
that the speaker hears him- or herself speaking with a lower- or higher-
pitched voice than they really have. These devices have less effect on
speech quality, and listeners hear the person sounding much more as
they sound under ordinary conditions. In both cases, stuttering is typically reduced or removed, although there are some people for whom
the devices have only minimal effect. For devices that alter the signal
and for devices that simply amplify it, people who stutter report that
they feel as if they are talking in chorus with another speaker, a circumstance known to enhance fluency.

There are two difficulties, aside from the cost, with these devices.
The first is that they are cumbersome and often odd in appearance. For
many individuals who stutter, the relief they get from stuttering is not
worth the embarrassment of wearing a device that makes them look
so different. The second problem is that the effect is not permanent
and may even wear off while the device is still being worn. Invariably,
when the device is removed the person begins to stutter again just as
before. Some of the manufacturers will try to convince potential customers that there are long-term benefits, but there is no evidence that
these devices are anything more than a prosthetic device that temporarily enables fluency.

Nevertheless, for some people (e.g., older clients who don't want
the trouble of therapy or who have not done well in therapy and don't
want to try again) who are willing to spend the money (the devices
tend to cost between $300 and $1,500) such a device may be an acceptable alternative. Similarly, school-age children who sometimes are
very difficult to treat may find some relief and better acceptance in

school through wearing such a device, although the fact that the device looks so unusual can be a powerful deterrent. Some devices can be attached to the telephone, making a readily available and invisible aid to this often dreaded speaking situation.

A well-trained speech clinician will be informed about these devices and will understand how and when to recommend a trial period for a client. Expense is something to be considered because the person who stutters typically does not continue to use the device for a very long time; many people just get tired of wearing them. Others find the techniques learned in therapy more portable, more permanent, and, of course, invisible.

Drug Therapies

In the only comprehensive review of research on the use of drugs in alleviating stuttering, Brady (1995) reviewed research on six different types of drugs studied over the last 30 years. He concluded that the "therapeutic benefits reported with all the above pharmacologic agents are modest at this time. Much clinical research needs to be done" (p. 510). The good news is that there has been a recent increase in efforts in this area. Currently, the large number of apparent breakthroughs have all turned out to be false in that the drugs did not really do very much, or there were permanent and unacceptable side effects.

One drug currently being researched is botulinum toxin (Stager & Siren, 1995). In large quantities, this drug is a lethal substance that has the effect of paralyzing muscles. When injected in a very small dose directly into one of the two vocal folds, it partially or completely paralyzes it, leaving the person with a hoarse-sounding but usable voice. In some cases, the vocal quality is unacceptable; one client reported sounding like Mickey Mouse for 3 months (P. Ramig, personal communication, June 14, 1995). In a person who stutters, this change often promotes more fluent speech. After several months, the effect wears off, and the person has to go back and get another injection. Clearly an invasive technique, and with yet unknown side effects (over time, the poison is absorbed into the body, and it is not known what the long-term effects of this may be), it is definitely not recommended by the researchers as a viable form of treatment, although some physicians, in what seems like callous disregard for their clients' welfare, will prescribe it.

Tranquilizing drugs and antidepressants have been studied, and, in some cases, some partial and/or temporary effects have been reported. Speech clinicians familiar with this literature can refer appropriate clients to a knowledgeable physician. However, it should be made clear to the client that such treatments are only experimental. Also there is really no evidence that drug treatments should replace regular therapy. At best, they are a supplement to speech therapy. Many clients seem to be helped by drug treatment when, in fact, the placebo effect is occurring. After a while, this wears off and the person is back where he or she started, having perhaps wasted a lot of time and money.

Listening Effects on Stuttering and Listener Reactions

One of the most striking effects on stuttering is that of the accepting listener. When a situation is created in which it is all right for a person to stutter, that is, when the stuttering will be completely accepted, it disappears or diminishes. A brief story will illustrate this. A young man who worked in a medical setting was interested in trying a drug that had been rumored to help alleviate stuttering. The clinician agreed to this but suggested that the effect should be documented. Arrangements were made to videotape the man before and after the dose was administered. When the tape was turned on and the young man was asked to describe his work, he started to talk with perfect fluency, even though he had not yet taken the drug. It was the first time the clinician had ever heard this person speak in any way but with the most severe stuttering. In spite of many attempts to make the situation more difficult for him, the man continued to speak fluently as long as the camera was recording him because he knew that in that situation there was no point in trying not to stutter. His stuttering was desirable at that moment.

Such dramatic effects teach us the power of the listener. The person who is not afraid to show his or her stuttering often achieves speech that is considerably more fluent than those who fear the judgment of listeners. This is why most individuals who stutter are far more fluent when talking to their speech therapist than they are when talking to other people. There is no reason to hide the stuttering and, in most cases, the client believes that the clinician accepts him or her in spite of the stuttering.

Listening is a great gift that the "normally nonfluent" can give to the person who stutters. Most individuals who stutter have a long history of not having been listened to completely. Too many times, people have heard only the stuttering and not the story behind it. Many people may have tried to help but in inappropriate, unhelpful ways (e.g., finishing sentences, giving advice such as slow down, etc.).

These listening effects can be turned to good advantage if people who stutter can learn to teach their listeners how to listen in a way that promotes fluency in the speaker. First, they can become more knowledgeable about the disorder of stuttering. Listeners who understand more about stuttering are easier to talk to. Second, listeners can become more familiar with the particular person's pattern of stuttering. When there are appropriate opportunities, the speaker can explain about good days/bad days, the effect of noise in the background, or any other aspect of his or her own particular way of stuttering. Just "advertising" the stuttering—that is, commenting on it, making it more obvious that *stuttering* is the problem at hand, not anxiety, ignorance, or a faulty memory—is helpful. Most listeners are genuinely interested in being helpful and will respond accordingly. Because it is well known that listeners stop paying attention to stuttering once they become more familiar with it, just talking more to any listener will result in the person who stutters paying less attention to the stuttering and more to the content. All are ways to educate the listener to be more accepting of stuttering.

In almost all circumstances, it is also helpful to be as direct and honest as possible about stuttering. A brief story will illustrate this. The senior author worked with a 12-year-old boy who reported at one session that he was nervous because his grandmother was coming for a visit. When asked, he volunteered that she often commented to his mother on the state of his stuttering—he was improving, he was having a setback, etc.—so that he could hear it. He felt that she listened only to the way he talked and not to what he was saying. He was advised to tell her how he felt and to express to her that he wanted to talk to her and have her listen to him. This kind of directness was a bit challenging for a 12-year-old, but he was a courageous kid and he did it. His grandmother listened and heard him. Things changed quickly. The grandmother stopped making comments, and the grandson stopped dreading her visits.

Paradoxes

Stuttering is a disorder of paradoxes,[5] of which the most important is the one that has to do with control. The more the person who stutters tries to control stuttering, the less control he or she actually has over it. Many such individuals are able, with great concentration, to speak fluently for a while, but exerting this kind of control is typically an exhausting proposition that cannot be sustained, and, in the end, the person returns to the original behavior with a sense of relief, often mixed with despair. Similarly, stuttering can disappear quite spontaneously, when, as in the story told previously, efforts to control it are abandoned. This is the principle of *letting go*.

Many people who stutter have discovered that if they can let go of their stuttering, that is, just let it happen and give up trying to control it, they can speak more freely and in fact stutter much less. So much of the behaviors we call stuttering are actually attempts to control, hide, or avoid it; when these are given up, the person's speech is much easier and less speech time is devoted to extraneous behaviors. Many individuals discover this fact on their own, usually after they have become adults and after many years of struggle. This principle is so strong in recovery from stuttering that the National Stuttering Project's monthly newsletter is called *Letting Go*. It is a basic principle of recovery. In letting go of the behavior, it is most helpful also to stop trying to avoid the feelings of fear, shame, anger, and let them happen. The person who stutters discovers that, by accepting and letting these feelings happen, they lose their power to control the person's behavior. Speech clinicians, parents, and friends can help people who stutter learn the principle of letting go by giving them opportunities to discover the value of this new way of thinking about stuttering and the feelings that accompany it.

Most people who stutter respond to the feeling that they are about to stutter by trying to hide, minimize, avoid, or escape from the behavior. As a result, they can never learn that stuttering is something they can do and survive. Speech clinicians and others can help them by supporting attempts to let the stuttering happen and realize that the consequences of it are an experience from which they all can learn and grow.

---

[5]Earlier, we described the paradoxes of stuttering derived from its recursion.

Adults who stutter have often internalized the reactions their parents had to them when they were stuttering as children. As a result, they may have adopted any one of a number of specific attitudes about their stuttering, including anxiety, shame, or anger. Speech clinicians and others can help the adult who stutters work through these feelings by listening nonjudgmentally and acknowledging the reality and the pain of these feelings. It is not helpful to tell adults who stutter that they shouldn't feel the way they do. The fact is, they *do* feel this way. Accepting the reality of their feelings, we have found, is the surest path to their dissolution.

The Process of Recovery

Many people who stutter have stopped stuttering, some with the help of speech therapy and some without such help. In these cases, themes of awareness and acceptance weave a common thread (Hood, 1974). This book's second author and other people recovering from stuttering date the beginning of their recovery to the time when they became willing to pay close attention to what they actually did when they stuttered; to what they felt before, during, and after the stuttering episodes; to identify and acknowledge their attitudes about their stuttering; and to begin to accept that the stuttering was a part of who they were—not something they could hide away in the closet.[6]

Many people who have recovered from stuttering reported substantial feelings of relief when they decided to stop fighting it and just go ahead and stutter. So many of the things they were doing in the attempt to minimize, hide, avoid, or escape from stuttering behavior had become incorporated into a pattern of struggle and avoidance that was a large part of their stuttering behaviors. Because so much of their behavior was based on the attempt to control their stuttering, giving up this control considerably reduced their stuttering behavior. This change in stuttering behavior then gave rise to new awarenesses, and the cycle continued.

What follows is a sketch of an approach that, though still in its infancy, has been implemented at the Temple University Stuttering

---

[6]The authors wish to acknowledge, with much gratitude, the work of 12-step author Melody Beattie (1990a; 1990b). The concepts of awareness, acceptance, and change are discussed frequently in her work *The Language of Letting Go.*

Center and is the philosophical basis upon which the Birch Tree Foundation was founded. As outlined in Figure 7.1, it combines elements of a traditional Van Riperian treatment, Gestalt experiential therapy, and principles of 12-step recovery programs. We see this ongoing cycle of awareness, acceptance, and change as a process of recovery.

Therapy as Conversation

For too long, speech therapy has been viewed as a hierarchical dyad, clinician and client, with the clinician in the superior, controlling role. We believe that the therapeutic framework must be broadened. Anne Wilson Schaef (1992) wrote eloquently of these problems with regard to psychotherapy. Like addiction, stuttering is a disorder of control. The person who stutters is trying to control a system (speech production) that has evolved so as to allow the speaker to relinquish close control. Although it is possible to control speech production for periods of time, this is not a normal way to speak, and it is extremely difficult, and impossible for many, to sustain this control of the uncontrollable for very long. Under such circumstances to relinquish some control to a speech clinician is confusing. People who stutter are often willing to be convinced that they can be taught how to control their speech, when, in our opinion, what they need to learn is to stop trying to control it so much. Many clinicians have bought into the idea that if the client would only exercise better control over his or her speech mechanism, he or she could speak without stuttering. We therefore believe that the speech clinician should not play the role of controller, that is, the giver of understanding and technique or the "professional" role. Instead, they should participate with the client in a process that will develop out of the client's own natural tendency to grow and change. For this reason, we believe that the hierarchical nature of stuttering therapy should be changed to one of mutual participation.

We call this process *conversation*, for a number of reasons. A conversation is, at its best, an ongoing exchange of information, opinions, ideas, definitions, perspectives, attitudes, and/or feelings between people. It does not have to be just two people, and, mediated by language, it is more than just an exchange of information. During the conversation, the participants develop and build up an idea that they have in common. In therapy for stuttering, the person who stutters has such an ongoing conversation via language with at least one other person. The other person is often a speech clinician, but not always. It may also be another person who stutters, or one's self, or a group of

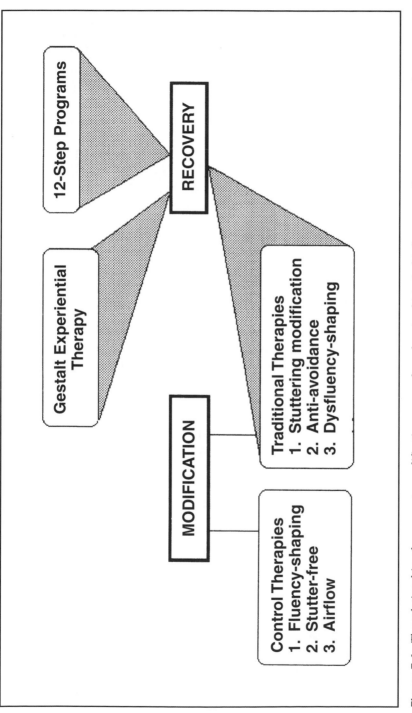

Figure 7.1. The relationship of recovery to modification approaches, showing historical influences on the recovery approach.

people. As a result of such a conversation, the recovery is a joint creation of the partners to the conversation. The word creation is used here in the same sense as it is used in art or music. Creation is a process that goes forward as a result of natural human tendencies, and it is only partially under the control of the artist. In therapy for stuttering, the process consists of the development of new awarenesses of stuttering behaviors and feelings and of other aspects of self, and of increased acceptance of one's stuttering and of one's self at the moment of stuttering. It also consists of changes in speech and other behaviors; beliefs about stuttering (or self); perceptions of self and others; attitudes toward stuttering, speech, and self; and feelings about stuttering, speech, listeners, or one's self. Just as two people having a conversation about politics or the beauty of autumn can gently create and develop in each other's minds a new, ongoing idea about these topics, so can a person who stutters and another person (or people) allow the former to develop in the direction of recovery from the burden that stuttering often is and toward the freedom of speech that is available, by right, to everyone.

Humans are social animals not meant to live in isolation. As such, we talk and listen to each other. We work and play together, celebrate and grieve together, create art for others to see, generate governments, and worship in company. We often try to "see the other's point of view." When willing, we can become educated through listening and connecting to the experiences of others. Most of our socializing consists of conversations in small groups of two or more. A conversation, again, is an ongoing exchange of ideas and feelings and an interaction in which the parties generate an idea and then build upon it until it becomes something new. It is an act of joint creativity, often a joyous and fulfilling enterprise. When people have a conversation about stuttering, their beliefs, perceptions, and thoughts about stuttering can, and almost certainly will, change. If one or more of those people is a person who stutters, the changes can be therapeutic. What follows is a brief summary of the distinction between recovery from stuttering and modification therapies.

The Difference Between Recovery from Stuttering and Modification Therapies

Previous therapies for stuttering have been based on modifying the behavior of people who stutter. There are two types of modification therapies: (a) those that teach the person controls he or she can use whenever talking (i.e., speech modification therapies or what have come to be called control therapies), and (b) those that modify the stuttering behavior itself in the direction of greater normality (i.e., stuttering modification therapies). Recovery is a different process, although it incorporates some principles of stuttering modification therapies.

Recovery is self directed; modification is other directed. Therapy for children is most effectively and efficiently done through modification because children are, by definition, not responsible for themselves; for adults, there is a choice. Many adults may want to rely on the techniques and processes of another person; for them, a modification approach may be best, although the more personal responsibility they can take, even in a modification approach, the more successful they will be. For those people who want to take on more of the responsibility, or who have more trust in their own processes, a recovery approach is, we believe, more effective and results in a more complete recovery, one that does not require constant monitoring of one's speech and with less chance of relapse.

In recovery, the person who wants to change is responsible for establishing the goals and choosing the experiences that will lead to achieving those goals. A clinician familiar with this kind of treatment can be of great help in suggesting goals and experiences that can be helpful, but the final authority for making these decisions rests with the stutterer.

Recovery is ongoing; modification has a beginning, middle, and end. At the beginning of modification therapy, goals are established. In the middle, work is done to achieve those goals. At the end, the achievement of the goals is assessed, processes for maintaining the goals are put in place, and then the process ends. In recovery, the process doesn't stop when the chosen goals are reached. Often likened to "a journey, not a destination," recovery continues. Unlike modification, it does not have a set of preestablished criteria for termination.

Recovery is a search for understanding that will be a foundation for change, not an attempt to change without the foundation. This may be the most important difference between recovery and modification. In recovery, the person tries to become more aware of who it is they are and what it is they do, to accept those aspects of themselves for the moment, and then, through increased awareness and acceptance, to discover that change happens with little or no effort. The foundation for change is thus the insights, altered perceptions, free flow of feelings, and awareness of attitudes. In recovery, change is seen as a process that will happen naturally unless barriers are placed in its way. The foundation for change removes those barriers by first helping the client become aware of and then accept the reality of them.

Recovery is a spiritual process. It is a journey one takes into one's self. Mich of the journey consists of removing the masks of denial and avoidance, learning to be honest with one's self, taking responsibility for one's self, and caring about one's self enough to be willing to bear the sometimes painful challenges of self-confrontation.

Recovery occurs in a linguistic domain. The changes that occur in recovery are mediated by language, by talking and listening in conversations with others. Although modification can also be mediated by language, it often minimizes language, and, in fact, language is unnecessary to the direct application of learning processes to the modification of behavior. This is not true for recovery, where the process occurs through a conversation.

Sources of the Recovery Approach

In addition to what we have pulled from various 12-step recovery programs, there is much that we are grateful for learning from other groups that are finding their way in a difficult world. We are grateful to the gay community for showing us the compelling need to be true to one's self. We are grateful to the African American community for showing us the importance of not accepting the stereotypical thinking of others, which serves only to "keep us in our place."

We are also grateful to both Charles Van Riper and Joseph Sheehan for saying the right things—but, unfortunately, at the wrong time. Forty years ago, it seems, people were more interested in quick fixes and external modification therapies. Today, we can look back on the last 40 years and see how most of the profession of speech pathology, as well as the people who stuttered, bought into the patently false notion that perfectly fluent speech is normal and desirable. In fact, it is neither normal nor desirable, and striving for it to the exclusion of other more important goals, either through the use of avoidance and denial or through therapies that try vainly to achieve perfect fluency, leads only to frustration and disappointment. Instead, clients and clinicians alike need to keep their eyes on the prize—freedom of speech, serenity and realizing one's full potential.

Step 1—Increasing Awareness

In the first stage, the person becomes increasingly aware of his or her stuttering behavior and of the feelings and thoughts that accompany it. The clinician or other supportive listener also becomes more aware of these behaviors, thoughts, and feelings. This increased awareness occurs as they discuss the details of specific stuttering events. The discussion can take place as these stuttering events happen. The partners can pause in the middle of a conversation about any topic to comment on the stuttering that just occurred. This is a very powerful tool because the event is fresh in the minds of both people, and the feelings of being frustrated, scared, and/or embarrassed still are present. Unpleasant emotions are often fleeting when they are stifled by the ready hand of denial.

It is also possible to reflect on past stuttering episodes. Although less compelling than events that have just occurred, events recalled from memory are often the only way to deal with stuttering that has happened in a person's life.

Two tools that are useful for enhancing the memory of events gathered from everyday life—current or past—are the tape recorder and the journal. The tape recorder brings back the acoustic events, more or less accurately, and this can help in refreshing memory and countering denial. The journal offers the opportunity to reflect honestly about what was felt at the time. Use of a journal is an invaluable tool in recovery.

The purpose of increasing awareness is twofold. First, it forms a substratum of common knowledge and understanding that makes continued conversations about stuttering more concrete. Awareness provides referents for the words of the conversation. Second, it is the primary weapon against denial. For most people who stutter, denial is the only defense immediately available against the psychological pain of the disorder, and it is sometimes necessary to tolerate some denial. Like sleeping, a person discovers that he or she has been in denial only through hindsight. There are many forms of denial, ranging from minimizing the problem to losing one's sense of presence (splitting, or *flying*) in the speech situation (see Chapter 3). Increased awareness counters this denial directly. The importance of a genuine feeling of safety cannot be overemphasized. If one thinks of denial as a warm coat against a cold chill, only as the environment warms up (i.e., becomes safe) is the person willing to remove the coat. So, it is important for the clinician to help create such a safe environment and wait patiently until the person feels safe enough in it to see the denial he or she was using.

Increasing Awareness of Behaviors

Perhaps the easiest place to start in the process of increasing awareness is with the behaviors. In addressing specific stuttering behaviors, it is useful to follow a three-part sequence of identify, locate, and characterize. A wide variety of research and clinical experience indicates that the following areas should be reviewed: the identification of stuttering and the client's definition of stuttering, the location of the behavior in the utterance, the distinction between normal and abnormal behavior, the anatomical focus of the stuttering behavior, the type of behavior, the intention of the behavior, the tempo and tension level of the behavior, the vocal pitch and quality during the behavior, the amount of force used in producing the sound, the sound/word on which the behavior occurs, the type of sentence the person is trying to say, the load of information on the word with which the stuttering behavior is associated, the listener, the speech situation, and the influence of a concomitant articulation or language disorder. The following series of questions are designed to initiate conversations that will increase awareness and understanding of these issues.

1. *Am I stuttering now or not?* This is the main issue for identifying when stuttering is happening, and it seems very simple. It isn't as simple as it appears, however. Each person creates a semantic space, an idea of what the word stuttering means for him or her, and the process of recovery will work best if this space is self-determined. In this way, the creation of recovery is truly the person who stutters' own process, rather than something imposed from the outside. As a person who stutters talks, there is often a point in the utterance where the person senses that soon, very soon, he or she is going to stutter, perhaps on that /p/ sound coming up. Then there may be a repetition of the /p/. But did the "stuttering" begin with the /p/, or did it begin with the anticipation of stuttering on the /p/? This is a problem of definition, as are all issues of identification. There is no right or wrong answer. If the person who stutters wants to define stuttering as including the anticipation, that is fine, and if he or she wants to keep the two things separate as different kinds of experience, that too is fine.

Similarly, an individual who stutters and who typically has hard vocal blockages may have a one-unit repetition—s-something like this. Is it stuttering or is it a kind of normal nonfluency, something any speaker might experience? The clinician might offer some general information by saying that one-unit repetitions are considered a normal type of nonfluency, although they are relatively rare in people who do not stutter. However, the decision about whether to consider this event as a stuttering behavior or as a normal nonfluency is up to the client, based on what it feels like to him or her. Again, by making this decision, the client takes personal responsibility for the decision of defining stuttering, a crucial element in developing the idea of recovery.

2. *Where in my body is this happening?* There is usually an anatomical location where the stuttering can be felt, a place where the muscles are tight or the air pressure high. Sometimes there are two places at the same time. There may be other accompanying sensations. Identifying these further defines the person's own individual experience of the disorder. This is one of those aspects of stuttering that is highly individualized. Some individuals usually block laryngeally and only occasionally, or never, block with their tongues or lips. Others have the exact opposite experience. A person who is covertly stuttering may have more difficulty in identifying the location(s) of the event(s) that constitute his or her stuttering, but once identified, this information will be very helpful in the process of recovery.

3. *What sound or word am I trying to say?* It is usually easy for a person who stutters to identify the troublesome sound or word because it looms large. At first, this is all that needs to be done. Each time the person stutters, he or she notes which sound or word prompts the stuttering. Some individuals seem more focused on the sound, others more on the word. Either is acceptable, but deciding is another step in taking ownership of the problem.

After a number of identifications in which the sound or word is identified, a pattern may or may not emerge. It may become clear that /b/ sounds are very often stuttered, or all fricative sounds (s, z, sh, ch, j), or words that refer to academic subjects, or specific words, or certain types of words. There is usually some kind of pattern for the adult who stutters. The patterns themselves are highly individualized (or there may be no pattern at all). Whether a pattern is identified or not, and, if so, what kind, is another piece of the larger picture of this particular person's stuttering. Completing this step of identification goes a little further in heightening self-awareness and helping the person take ownership of the problem.

4. *What is the purpose of my sentence?* Am I saying this sentence in order to convince, explain, state, ask, greet, say goodbye, tell a joke, share a thought or feeling, apologize, or confess a misdeed?

There are many, many purposes in uttering a sentence. Sometimes there is a pattern here as well. The person who stutters may have more trouble with questions, or with assertive statements of opinion, or attempts to convince, or in telling a joke. It may be that there is no such pattern; however, if there is, the nature of the pattern can be identified and added to the description of what stuttering means to this person.

5. *Where in the sentence is the stuttering located?* Although in general stuttering tends to occur more on the first three words of a sentence than in other locations, the pattern may be entirely different in any individual. Some individuals stutter toward the end of a sentence, others may stutter on words that carry a high load of information. An example can be seen in the following two sentences:

> The prince has not used the *coach* all year long.
>
> Six white horses pulled the golden *coach.*

Imagine a blank in place of the word *coach.* Most adult speakers of English would have little trouble supplying the word in the second sentence, but in the first sentence it would be difficult. The word coach carries a much higher load of information in the first sentence than in the second. There are a number of things that the prince may not have used all year. When it is easy to supply the missing word, it carries little additional information. For example in the sentence "Chicken cackle but ducks _____" it isn't necessary to write in the word at all. If you speak the language you know what word to use. Therefore, it carries no additional information.

For some people who stutter the load of information is an important variable in determining when their stuttering will occur. Discovering the relative importance of this variable in determining the location of the stuttering is yet another piece in the jigsaw puzzle for each person who stutters. As these pieces are identified and put in place, the individual nature of the person's stuttering behavior takes form. As each decision about this form is made, the person generates a personal meaning of the word stuttering.

6. *With whom am I talking?* For many individuals, the listener is an important variable affecting the severity of the stuttering, even whether or not it occurs. Many people who stutter report stuttering

more when they talk to groups, strangers, or authority figures, but the type of listener that is difficult (easy) to talk with is a highly individual matter (e.g., people in certain occupations, people with a certain appearance, or people in a certain role). Of course, specific people also may be identified as difficult (easy) listeners (e.g., spouse, parent, or uncle). This pattern, like many others, is highly individual, and identifying it helps to complete the picture.

7. *In what situation am I talking?* Perhaps the best known of the variables that can influence stuttering, the speech situation is a broad category that can include listeners, sentence types, and even words and sounds. We use it here more narrowly to refer to aspects of the circumstances under which a person is talking other than listeners, words, sounds, and sentence types. One person we knew had great difficulty saying numbers and, as a result, stuttered most severely when making long-distance telephone calls and buying tokens for the subway. For others, their most severe stuttering occurs when ordering in a restaurant, or in an argument, or ordering at a drive-up window intercom. These are just a few examples; there is an infinite number of difficult situations. Any situation in which a person has had a particularly difficult time in the past is likely to become a "difficult" situation. Identifying these unpleasant situations helps to complete the personal pattern of stuttering.

8. *Is my voice pitched higher or lower than usual or is the quality different (strained, hoarse, tense)?* This is just another possibility. As children, many people who stutter increase the pitch of their voices while repeating syllables or words in an almost siren-like quality. This pattern may be a simple vocal pattern of increasing muscular tension or it may be a learned strategy to change the parameters of vocal tract dynamics so as to escape from the episode. Either way, the adult needs to become aware of vocal changes, either as a result or a cause of stuttering, are part of his or her pattern.

Some children use a "baby voice" during episodes of repetition. Getting in touch with these "inner child" reactions to feelings of frustration or fear as an adult is an important first step in learning to deal with them.

9. *Is my articulation soft or hard? Am I saying a sound that has been a problem in the past (an articulation disorder or mispronunciation)?* For a substantial minority of children, stuttering is associated with attempts to correct an articulation disorder, with or without the aid of a speech therapist, or, in some cases, to meet models of perfect articulation that

parents or older siblings present. When children attempt to improve articulation, they often put too much muscular effort into the attempt. As this increased muscular effort becomes a part of their approach to the act of speaking, the stage is set for a habit of reaction that can lead to stuttering as an adult. When the adult becomes aware of this ancient pattern, he or she takes a step toward recovery.

10. *Is this behavior a repetition, prolongation, blockage, broken word, tremor, or a combination of these?* Part of the identification of each behavior at the moment it is occurring is its categorization by type. Question 10 provides the usual categories of *primary (nonreactive) behaviors,* but no one should assume that there is anything sacred about the list. Many systems of categorization have been offered. A good system should clearly differentiate among different types of behavior. For example, it makes sense to combine a three-unit repetition (li-li-li-like this) with a two-unit repetition (li-li-like this), considering the number of units a nonessential difference. Similarly, it makes sense to distinguish between repetitions and prolongations not only because they sound different, but because they are produced as a result of different kinds of movements in the vocal tract. Wingate's (1964) system is perhaps in widest use, but it does seem to be in error in calling prolonged silences "prolongations." We prefer to call these behaviors blockages and then specify their location, because they involve a very different physiological process.

Whatever system of categorization is used, the person who stutters can learn to differentiate among the various behaviors that he or she exhibits until it is possible to say, "That was a tremor" or "That was a vocal blockage" or "That was a repetition" with confidence. This process is important in two ways. First, learning to separate a complex phenomenon into its component parts with consistent labels for the parts provides anyone with a sense of mastery over the phenomenon. Second, it provides a language with which the phenomenon can be described, analyzed, and discussed. Although this also provides mastery, more importantly, it enables the conversation that client and clinician (or friend, parent, etc.) will have about the problem.

Question 10 also begins to touch on the increased acceptance that is so important in recovery. When the person who stutters says, "There, I prolonged the /s/ sound," he or she is taking ownership of the problem, is also saying "That is what I am doing now," and it is a bit closer to saying "I accept that what I am doing now is stuttering."

11. *Am I trying to force the word out; backing up; trying to get rhythmic support; postponing, avoiding, or hiding sounds, situations, subjects, or*

silences; substituting; or doing some other trick? The *secondary (reactive) behaviors* are used voluntarily (at least in the early stages) to deal in some way with the primary or nonreactive behaviors. The list given here in Question 11 is only partial and open ended. There is great and seemingly infinite variety in the ways that people who stutter can learn to deal with the behaviors that plague them. As a result, the identification of these behaviors is particularly important in filling out the picture of each individual's stuttering, of defining the word stuttering in the particular conversation that is taking place.

Often, it is not just the form of the reactive behaviors that is important, but the motivation behind them. One woman pursed her lips when she spoke. When she said that she did this in order to "make a channel" for the sound to come out, it was evident that she didn't really understand how the process of speech production worked, and it was also not surprising that the lip pursing did little to facilitate speaking. Much the same thing can be said for most reactive behaviors—they do not help, and often they hinder the process of speaking. Backing up and saying a sentence over again wastes valuable time and often leads to stuttering on words before the feared word, thus compounding the problem. Postponing only wastes time. Pushing and forcing seem only to make the vocal folds lock more tightly together in a Valsalva maneuver. "Straining" the voice to make it hoarse may increase fluency a little, but it reduces energy, weakens communication, and may damage the vocal folds. A discussion of these motivations and an examination of their actual utility is an important step in increasing the awareness of both the person who stutters and the conversational partner. It is important for the clinician (or other conversational partner) not to take issue with the client in these circumstances. If a client changes words and feels that not doing so will increase the chances of stuttering, and if he or she is not willing to take such a risk yet, there is no value in trying to argue the point. The partner needs also to be accepting. When the time is right, the client will see the nonutility of a behavior and will give it up.

12. *Is this behavior struggled or easy? Is it rapid or slow in tempo?* These two questions are similar because the struggle to get out of a stuttering episode often takes the form of trying to go faster. Talking rapidly is associated with increased muscle tension, so the act of trying to talk faster simply makes matters worse. It is, however, a natural response to the feeling of being stuck or stopped in one's tracks. Becoming aware of this struggle, in whatever form it takes, is an important early step. Struggling to talk is a self-defeating,

self-sabotaging behavior. Typically, this strategy was adopted in the person's earliest years of stuttering, perhaps when he or she was 3 or 4 years old. A child at this age who feels stuck has no way of dealing with the experience except to struggle. We have all seen toddlers trying to accomplish some task, such as pulling a toy, that is simple for an adult. The toy gets stuck on the leg of a chair. The adult can see that all the child has to do is stop pulling, go back to the toy, and pull it out from behind the chair leg. But the toddler yanks and pulls to make the toy come along, getting increasingly frustrated. Sometimes, the child stops and sees the solution; sometimes he or she just cries. For the very young person who stutters and is trying to talk, an episode of repeated words or syllables is a similar experience. He or she wants to talk, but there is a sudden obstacle to accomplishing this goal. The child pushes, but nothing happens. He or she pushes harder, triggering vocal reflexes that only jam the speech mechanism harder in its stuck place. Frustration results. Some children stop, consider, and perhaps ease their way out of the moment. These children are not likely to develop chronic stuttering. Others cannot deal with the frustration in such a calm way. They may panic, dissolve into tears of anger, give up, or say something else. At this moment, they begin to learn a pattern of avoidance, inner rage, or sadness.

Few things are more useful for the adult who stutters than getting in touch with the childlike reactions that may still be interfering with the ability to talk. Being aware of these feelings is the first step in seeing their nonutility. The problem is one of dealing, as an adult, with the child that is still within us. Awareness of the situation is a first step.

Increasing Awareness of Thoughts

Our thoughts, or cognitions, are (a) a collection of beliefs taught to us by others, (b) our perceptions of the world based on those beliefs, and (c) our attitudes toward life that spring from our perceptions. For example, problematic beliefs might include "I am not a good speaker;" "Stuttering is shameful;" "If only I didn't stutter, I could . . . ." Problematic perceptions might include "People think I am nervous or crazy;" "No one is listening to me;" "Everyone is laughing at me." Problematic attitudes might include "I must never let my stuttering show."

These and other thoughts can occur in anyone who stutters. Most often the thoughts occur during stuttering, but sometimes thoughts occur before and after stuttering, as in anticipations and retrospections. Examples of *anticipations* include "I am going to stutter in just a second" or "Uh oh, here comes an /s/ word." Examples of *retrospections* include "I was really stuck just then" or "That wasn't as bad as I thought it would be."

Some thoughts are repetitive and intrusive; others occur only once and are not particularly important. Whatever thoughts occur are part of the pattern of stuttering in an individual, and discovering what they are and being aware of them as they occur helps to build a sense of who the client is. Some of these thoughts can have substantial power. The anticipation of stuttering can trigger stuttering, and a morbid retrospection of a previous conversation can disturb one's present thinking.

Beliefs have a powerful effect. A belief such as "I am not a good speaker" can rob the person who stutters of the gratification he or she might otherwise feel from an intimate exchange or from a valuable contribution to a business meeting. Similarly, the individual who believes that stuttering is shameful creates the mechanism for a deeply punitive response to every stuttering episode that erodes his or her sense of self-worth.

Perceptions alter the way a person processes input from others. A person who stutters and who perceives impatience in his or her listeners will often try to speed up. One who perceives anger may feel afraid or perhaps belligerent. Perceptions, which are derived from beliefs, are a kind of filter that allows us to make sense of our experiences. As a filter, however, they can prevent people from seeing the true value of their contributions to a conversation, and they can twist social relations in a way that makes it difficult to maintain friends. The person who stutters and perceives that others believe him or her to be stupid because of the stuttering may try to create a show of intelligence, reducing spontaneity and self-expression. In this and many other ways, stuttering makes a person be someone other than who he or she really is. It is one of the great tragedies of this disorder.

Attitudes could be considered a filter of what goes out, just as perceptions are a filter of what comes in. The person whose attitude is that stuttering is the worst thing he or she could do will not allow the stuttering to show and may be willing to do many things, even very abnormal ones, rather than stutter. Of course, such an attitude opens the door to acquiring many abnormalities on top of the preexisting stuttering behaviors.

When shared with a clinician or another supportive conversational partner, these thoughts should be acknowledged as part of the person's pattern. Usually, an individual's way of stuttering has evolved over a period of time, and the rediscovery and telling of their story is a powerful part of the conversation that is therapy. The story of a person who stutters is the tale of who he or she has become as a result of the disorder. It defines the person insofar as stuttering has determined him or her.

Increasing Awareness of Emotions

Emotions are neither good nor bad. They just are. Identifying emotion (or other feelings, both physical and psychological) is a surprisingly difficult step for many people who stutter. A person with severe stuttering encounters substantial psychological pain every day, and it becomes necessary to adopt defenses against it. Denying the feelings or turning them off is one defense that develops in people who stutter. Emotionally shut down for so long, these individuals may have learned to deny and ignore their feelings. Other people may have evolved a way of not being present during the stuttering. Their minds protect them by establishing another reality where the pain doesn't exist or is muted. Whenever the stuttering occurs, they momentarily escape to this "other place." It is an understandable defense against the pain, but, of course, it does not help in finding solutions. The pain often finds a way in anyway.

Under circumstances such as these, it is not surprising that people who stutter often seem not to know what they are feeling at the moment they stutter. It may be helpful to prompt them with the ever popular "mad, glad, sad, hurt, or afraid: pick one!" A more inclusive list also includes shame, embarrassment, pain, humiliation, insecurity, and frustration. In this first step, it is necessary only to identify the feeling and acknowledge its existence, remembering, again, that feelings are not good or bad; they just are. They need to be owned and honored. It is important that the feeling is fully experienced and not attenuated by defensive reactions, but this step cannot be rushed.

Two tools are imperative in the process of recovery—sharing and honesty. Both are necessary, neither is sufficient. Sharing is putting our experiences into words and letting someone else know about them.[7]

---

[7]Although words are most commonly used, drawing (artwork), music, or any art form can all be forms of sharing if they are the means by which the individual makes him- or herself known to another.

As soon as an inner experience is shared, it becomes more real to the person; language puts our experiences out where we can deal with them and where we will be less likely to push them aside. Different forms of sharing include conversations (with another) and journaling (a written conversation with one's self).

Honesty is the tool that enables genuine, authentic sharing. When an individual is still hiding behind denial, sharing will be incomplete. Denial does serve a purpose in the earliest stages of recovery, protecting the person from experiences that he or she is not yet ready to have. When it is safe, the person can be more vulnerable. The process of recovery is one that occurs with other people. Frequently, people's fears are so deeply ingrained that, without support and help, they continue to "run back for cover." It has been said that life is a package deal. People must be willing to face the whole picture (painful parts included) in order to see what options are available. Being honest about themselves to themselves and with others is an important ingredient. It is often said that secrets make us sick. Sharing and honesty expose those secrets and allow the individual to begin to heal.

A quintessential question is "What are you feeling right now?" It begins a conversation about the present feeling and focuses the client on the present. As a result of their many painful experiences with stuttering, many clients are not in very good touch with their feelings. For others, the sharing of feelings is itself frightening, unfamiliar, or awkward. In these circumstances, it is helpful to begin with something that is easier or less threatening. For example, the conversational partner (e.g, a clinician) might ask, "Can you feel your toes inside your shoes, the pressure of your back against the chair, or your stomach, head, or heart?" These physical sensations can be explored and described, and, in time, it will be easier to say, "I feel afraid." A number of similar questions, all elaborations on the same theme, could be used: "How do you feel now about the experience that you had yesterday (last week, etc.)?" "How do you feel about the experience that you are going to have tomorrow (next week, etc.)?"

An important tool in this work is paying attention. Speech goes by very fast, and the feelings that accompany it can also be transient. Denial is often whispering in the ear: "You don't need to pay attention to that; it probably won't be pleasant." As a person who stutters begins to get over denial, it will become easier to pay attention to what is happening before, during, and after an episode of stuttering. There are many things to notice. One's feelings, physical and emotional, before, during, and after a speech situation in which stuttering is anticipated may be helpful to check. Similarly, an adult who stutters may have emotions about some of his or her childhood experiences, or about something that happened just last week, that are critical in discovering who he or she is right now.

Step 2—Becoming More Accepting of One's Self at the Moment of Stuttering

The second stage is accepting each awareness (i.e., some aspect of the stuttering) for what it is *at the moment*. Often, the initial reaction to this new awareness is resistance or a need to eliminate the unwanted behavior through sheer will power. For example, with regard to a particularly offensive secondary behavior, the person may swear that he or she will not do it any more. This reliance on will power usually backfires. Will power is like a parent telling a child that he or she must do something. It may get the job done, but frequently there is resentment and anger at the instructions, even if the person has been successful. If the child hasn't been successful, there will be guilt and shame. With encouragement and support, an individual can learn to accept the behavior for what it is at the moment. He or she can learn not to struggle with it, to let it go. It is important to remember that acceptance is not approval. It is not an attempt to turn clients into "happy stutterers." It is a countering weapon against the defensive reactions of avoidance, fear, and struggle. There are many areas where acceptance is important, including acceptance of behaviors, attitudes, and feelings. The ability to fully accept one's feeling of shame regarding stuttering can be for some a defining moment when the stutter begins to lose its grip.

At the behavioral level, self-acceptance means accepting the reality of stuttering behaviors. If a person has stuttered, that is what he or she has done—repeated sounds, blocked on vocalization, exhaled to change the dynamics of voicing, backed up to get a running start, and so forth. There is no substitute for accepting reality, but this acceptance is not done in a condemnatory way. It is not a matter of angrily saying, "'There, I have gone and messed up again." Rather, it is a matter of calmly accepting the reality of that moment. It does not mean accepting that one is going to stutter forever. Given the reality that many people have recovered from stuttering, that belief may be unrealistic. Acceptance means simply surrendering to the current reality.

For the moment, the person realizes that he or she is powerless to control the events that are occurring.

There is relief in this surrender. It isn't necessary to try to regain control. The episode will end and life (and speech) will go on. Once stuttering is happening, accepting that fact is the surest and quickest route to allowing the tense, stiffened, or trembling muscles to return to a more comfortable level of relaxation. It may help to trust that the speech mechanism knows what it is doing, as indeed it does.

It is the same with thoughts and feelings. They are what they are. For example, once a person is aware that he or she is having a morbid anticipation of stuttering on an upcoming word, or a feeling of dread, these feelings can be accepted. Trying to shake them off, ignore them, or shout them down will lead only to additionally extraneous thoughts and behaviors that will further complicate the stuttering pattern. In this approach to treatment, simplicity is the goal. People who stutter often pick up a lot of baggage as they go through life, acquiring a little head movement here, a habit of reflecting on past dysfluencies there, and so on, until they are carrying an enormous load; they are weighing down the fleeting and airy process of speech with a sackful of impedimenta. Trying to think different thoughts or feel different feelings only puts another chunk of stuff in the sack. Accepting the thoughts and feelings for what they are turns the sack over and empties it out on the ground, where it can stay as the person walks away.

Behaviors, thoughts, and feelings are all part of what constitutes a human being. As previously stated, stuttering takes people off the path of who they are becoming and sends them down a dark and rocky way. On that path they become self-denying, self-defeating, and sometimes self-destructive—strangers to themselves. Self-acceptance starts them down the road to knowing the strength and beauty that all individuals have. With self-acceptance, they stay on the path, in touch with who they really are.

Step 3—Change

The third stage is change, or "Getting out of the way." Once people who stutter are aware of their problem and accept it for what it is, there are many ways than can and do change. They can learn that there are better ways of being dysfluent and reacting to dysfluencies. Some are less noticeable, less painful, or less full of effort than others. They can learn about the process of making speech sounds and use those processes to make speech happen. "Trying not to stutter" doesn't work. The effort to change in this way is misplaced and will result in more baggage, not less. The process of change instead is one of getting out of the way and letting one's self talk. Often, perhaps, always, it is more than speech that is allowed to happen. Stuttering can and often does change people in more profound and broader ways, making them angry at listeners or afraid of certain types of people. These different ways of being will also slip away as they are first made more conscious and then are accepted for what they are. The person who is underneath the stuttering-engendered reactions then can come out and be who he or she really is.

Some useful techniques that people who stutter might want to adopt include the following:

Repairing

(See Chapter 6 for a description.) Essentially, repairing means using behaviors that will produce forward-moving speech sounds instead of behaviors that result in blockage or repetition. At the behavioral level, it is simply learning to talk instead of stutter.

Letting It Out

Like getting out of the way, letting the words come out is a proactive technique that replaces struggling. It works more on a feeling level than on a behavioral one. It is helpful to imagine that the words are like children lined up and waiting to go out to recess. They want to go out. When a person stutters, it is as though the kid at the end of the line got pushed, and, as a result, the whole line falls down, blocking the door. Just let words go out; that is their natural direction. Although, of course, words themselves do not have the desire to be spoken, in reality the process of producing words is semiautomatic and does not require very much attention or effort on the speaker's part. From the speaker's perspective, it *feels* as though the words "want" to come out. Letting them out means an abandonment of all the struggling, forcing, and pushing that so often characterizes the speech of people who stutter.

Giving Oneself the Necessary Time

Stuttering uses up time without adding information to the utterance, creating a kind of time deficit. The person who stutters may feel as though he or she is always behind. The culture has a kind of standard that says that information should flow at a certain rate. When stuttering occurs, it breaks this standard, leaving the person with the feeling that he or she is behind schedule. The person then tries to talk very fast to catch up. Sometimes this very rapid speech actually makes him or her more fluent because the mechanism is loosened and muscle tension reduced. However, rapid speech more typically increases muscle tension and makes the person's speech less fluent. The attempt to make up the time that stuttering behaviors have lost thus can create time pressure and more stuttering behaviors.

There are also many sources of time pressure that are just a part of everyday life, from ordering in a fast-food restaurant when there is a waiting line to saying one's name in an introduction, where even a slight hesitation makes one look foolish. We all live in time pressure. For the stutterer, whose disorder creates additional time pressure, the sources of time pressure external to the stuttering only make matters worse. Time pressure in its many forms is probably the most potent disrupter of speech for the person who stutters.

Furthermore, if a person is trying new ways of talking, feeling, and thinking, these are never as automatic as the old familiar ones, and it often feels to the person that the use of every new behavior is using up time. The reality may well be the opposite, but because the old way is automatic and requires less thought, it seems to go by more quickly. This is another reason why increased awareness promotes fluency. As the person feels everything that is happening during speech, his or her sense of time passing becomes more accurate. With this awareness, the time taken up by the new behavior will be more realistically assessed.

How much time does a person have for talking? Hard as it may be, we need not feel obligated to match cultural norms if they are unrealistic for us. Each of us has a right to the time we need for communication. This most human of activities takes time, and it takes whatever time is required. No one would argue that a person in a wheelchair has a right to as much time as necessary to get across the road before traffic begins to whizz by. So it is with speech. The person with normally fluent speech who has trouble finding the right words to say may require more time to express thoughts and feelings. The person who has more to say, or who has a more complicated idea to share, requires more time as well. It is no different for the person who stutters. He or she may need more time because of the stuttering, or for any other reason. It doesn't matter. We are all entitled to the time we need to communicate, which is a basic human right.

Basic as it is, others do not always give us the time we need. They may interrupt. They may finish sentences. They may be rude, misguided, or nervous themselves. In any event, it is not their business to decide how much time we need. It is our business to grant to ourselves the time we need to say what we have to say. People who stutter can work to accept that they are entitled to talking time.

Saying What One Wants

Just as we are entitled to time, we are also entitled to say what we want. Many people who stutter learn to change words as a way of being more fluent, or they learn to stay away from certain topics, or they order in a restaurant what they can say rather than what they want to eat. These are all forms of denying self, of putting fluency first. It is an other way of walking down that dark and rocky path that takes us away from who we really are. For the person who stutters, changing a word may seem like a tiny sacrifice in order not to be embarrassed or humiliated, and, if that is where a person is at the moment, it can be accepted for the reality it is. In a similar way, it may seem trivial to order string beans instead of carrots because "string beans" can be said more easily. What one wants to eat is, however, a part of who one is at that moment. Although each word that is changed may seem insignificant, these words accumulate, leaving the person feeling unfulfilled and noncommunicative. These forms of avoidance are, in a sense, dishonest.

Telling Listeners What One Needs Them to Do

Many listeners, out of nervousness or discomfort, finish sentences for people who stutter, lose eye contact with them, or say something such as "Just take it easy, relax, I'm in no hurry." Generally, these reactions are not helpful, although they may be well intended. Most people who stutter don't like them and wish that the listener would simply listen. It can be very helpful to work toward developing an attitude of managing one's listeners. If the person who stutters doesn't want them to finish sentences, he or she can tell them so, with respect and even with understanding of their good intentions.

Many people who stutter give their power away to their listeners: "The listener will think I'm stupid so I must do whatever I can not to stutter." This is letting the listener and his or her reactions be in control over the speech of the person who stutters. There are other ways that people who stutter give their power away to listeners. The second author remembers how the speed of the listener's speech influenced her own stuttering behavior. If the person with whom she was having a conversation was a fast talker, she felt the pressure to talk as fast, and this increased her own sense of time pressure. Another person often found herself acutely aware that the listener was made nervous by her stuttering, and she tried hard (too hard) not to stutter to "rescue" the listener from this anxiety. Most of the time, these situations come down to worrying too much about what the listener will think if one stutters. People who stutter can work to remember that they have more power than they may realize, and that it doesn't help to give that power away to the listeners.

We have known for some time that listeners actually hear the stuttering less as they become more used to it. As with many things, just hearing a lot of stuttering makes it seem more familiar and comfortable. Those who have known people who stutter for a long time report that they hardly hear it all, and speech therapists who work with these individuals report that they sometimes find it hard to hear the stuttering because they have come to see beyond the person's stuttering. Thus, one way that a person who stutters can manage his or her listeners is simply *by talking more* to them. The more the listener hears, the sooner the feeling of discomfort and nervousness will fade, and they will hear the stuttering less and less. They will be attending more to the content and less to the form.

Being Open About Stuttering

Of course, being open about stuttering helps also. One of the reasons that listeners are uncomfortable with stuttering is that they don't know what is happening. This is particularly true when the person who stutters has adopted methods for hiding the stuttering. One young man had a way of drawing out his vowels in a kind of singsong pattern and filling what would otherwise have been stuttering with many throwaway phrases, such as "Oh, yes, I see"; "Hmm"; repeating a just-said phrase; and "Yes, OK." All of these phrases were delivered in the singsong manner. There was still some stuttering, but most of it was covered up with all the extraneous verbiage. Needless to say listeners thought this young man very odd. To them, he was an eccentric person to whom it was difficult to listen. Many didn't even know he had a stuttering problem, which was his original purpose in adopting his strange way of talking. Although they didn't think he stuttered, many listeners may well have thought much worse—that he was crazy or just "weird." By learning how to be more open about his stuttering, he put everyone at ease, found himself in more direct contact with people, and was able to communicate far more effectively than he had in the past, even though he still stuttered at that stage. He was soon able to address the stuttering itself. Before he had learned to be open about the stuttering, there really wasn't very much stuttering on which to work. At the time of this writing, his entire speech pattern was much improved and he was starting to feel more in touch with himself.

Helpful Hints for the Process of Change

Change is often frightening and uncomfortable; thus, as changes begin to occur, it is important to cycle back through the first or second steps and describe once again the feelings associated with the experience of change. An important idea to counter this fear of change is the suggestion that the person can "trust the process." This means that the person realizes that he or she is afraid, becomes fully aware of that feeling, but has enough faith in the process to allow the change to happen anyway. "Feel the fear and do it anyway" is also a helpful slogan.

An important kind of trust for people who stutter is trusting their own speech mechanism. With countless experiences of having been betrayed by an uncontrollable, errant mouth, tongue, or larynx, it is to be expected that the person will find it difficult to trust his or her own speech mechanism. Yet, the process of producing speech sounds is a mechanical one. If the mouth moves in a certain way, the flow of air is present, and the vocal cords are configured appropriately, the expected sounds will occur. After having had an explanation of how these things work, the person who stutters can be helped by learning to trust that the speech mechanism is going to do what it is going to do. Perhaps it will bounce around a little or freeze momentarily. Such things are beyond control. But if the flow of air is maintained, the vocal cords adjusted, and the movements of the mouth slow and purposeful, the sound will be produced.

Another useful slogan is "Keep coming back." Whenever something new is being tried—whether it is a new behavior or a new way of thinking or feeling about stuttering, speech, or listeners—it is to be expected that the person from time to time will forget, slip, or just not do what has been suggested. If the clinician has made this new way of doing or thinking an "assignment" that "should" be done, clients are going to feel manipulated or pressured into doing it. When the slip occurs, they will feel guilty. They have "failed," "not done what they ought to have done or done what they ought not to have done," or "sinned." It doesn't have to be a clinician who has set them up in this way. People set themselves up for guilt in just the same way by saying "I should do this" "I shouldn't do that" "If only I could try harder to . . . ." As a result, when they don't do what they have told themselves they "should" do, in the most human of all responses, they feel disappointed in themselves or guilty. These reactions are unpleasant and painful, and to avoid them, people will increase their resistance, be less inclined to try, and consequently fail even more. This downward spiral is often at the heart of relapse, a complete reversion to old ways of thinking, feeling, and talking. It is a loss of trust in the process.

The clinician (or the client, friend, or parent as clinician) can suggest that new ways of talking, thinking, and feeling can be tried as an experiment. If the attempt doesn't work, the client can simply "come back" to it. If it doesn't work again, or the client forgets to do something, he or she can just keep coming back. The phrase "Keep coming back" is the opposite of "You should do this." When told what we should do, the child in us resents being forced, may sabotage the attempt, and, if it succeeds, will still be angry about it. If it fails, our "child" will feel guilty. The idea of keep coming back means instead that the client tries something, not as an obligation, but as an experiment, with the joy of curiosity and the excitement of adventure. If the experiment fails, it can be tried again with the same sense of adventure. If it succeeds, it is something that the person has done for him- or herself, not something performed out of a sense of obligation or as a result of coercion.

The Spiritual Foundation of Recovery

When a person engages in therapy, he or she is in a creative, spiritual process. By spiritual, we don't mean anything religious. Rather, we refer to the processes of growth and becoming that are a part of life for everyone. We begin as infants, with certain genetic proclivities, a level of energy that is often too much for our parents to handle, and an entire world to learn about. Our parents present parts of that world to us, and we grow to fit that picture. If the family is dysfunctional, through substance abuse, sexual abuse, or neglect, we will adopt dysfunctional ways of being. These are ways to survive in a dysfunctional family, but they take that child away from who he or she might otherwise become.

It is the same with stuttering. Being unable to communicate easily with one's parents, siblings, and friends interferes with the natural social intercourse that is the medium by which we all grow into our adult selves. In addition, it is frustrating and sometimes frightening. Often, parents don't know what to do or are misguided and make a number of mistakes. Even the most ideal of parents make mistakes, and it is not surprising that, given a baffling and frustrating problem like stuttering, some parents might make more mistakes than usual. Having a child who has a problem is difficult; it makes parents doubt their instincts. They suddenly don't know what to do. The effects of this confusion and uncertainty on the child who stutters can only be imagined. In any event, these effects are unique to each child and his or her family circumstances.

When recovery is viewed as a "spiritual" journey, it means that the person finds his or her way back to the original path. People who find recovery return to the essence of their being.

Some questions that can initiate conversations that focus on the spiritual aspect of recovery include the following:

> Who am I?
>
> How do I introduce myself?
>
> On what roles do I key my identity?
>
> What do I think/fear might happen if these roles were taken away—or if I couldn't tell anyone?
>
> What do I really like about myself? Why?
>
> What would I really like to change about myself, if I could?
>
> What masks have I developed that I hide behind?
>
> How do I give my power away to my listeners?

The answers to these questions will be long and complicated, developed in conversations that will be unique to each individual. And, they will change as the person changes.

Not a Formula

The three stages of recovery—awareness, acceptance, and change—are not a one, two, three formula for therapy. They are performed over and over again for different behaviors, thoughts, and feelings as they occur. They are consequently more like a cycle of recurring steps at different levels of recovery. Figure 7.2 illustrates this idea. The partner or clinician's role in this recurring cycle is that of conversationalist. A conversation is a way to develop an idea through the use of language. Therapy takes place in the domain of language, and the ideas developed are helpful to the person trying to recover (Anderson & Goolishian, 1988). Both parties create and form these ideas as they develop new awareness, concepts, and beliefs, or as they alter old ones. As ideas change and develop, the words used to describe them will also change. The ideas developed in this conversation relate to, in fact they *are,* the client's ongoing recovery.

The partner/clinician also is changed by the conversation. Primarily, this change occurs in the clinician's understanding of the client and of the client's stuttering. However, as this happens, the clinician's more general understanding of what stuttering is will also change. Both parties to this therapeutic conversation are finding their way.

Therapy is essentially a creative process, whether it is seen as an art form, a scientific endeavor, or some combination of both. In the creative process, a person finds something of him- or herself and represents it in some way, then makes it available to others. Just as a painter

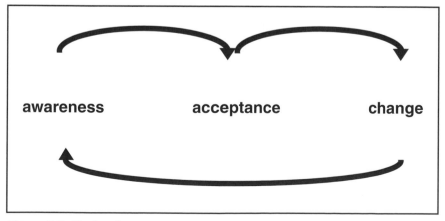

Figure 7.2. Cycles of recovery.

sets down something of him- or herself on canvas, then shows it to people, therapy is the art of finding aspects of one's self and then using them in front of other people. Recovery is a process that occurs in the client as a result of insights and learning that the client acquires. It may certainly be facilitated by interaction with a clinician or someone else, but it is not the interaction itself, although it may seem that way. Recovery is a word that describes the change that happens in the client.

In therapy, as in art, there is self-expression, a willingness to risk, and a sharing of the result (Zinker, 1977). Writing about Gestalt psychotherapy, Joseph Zinker stated what is true of all therapy:

> [It] is permission to be exuberant, to have gladness, to play with the nicest possibilities for ourselves within our short lives. For me it stands for all that is in front of me, for all that promises completeness of experiencing, for the things to come which are awesome, frightening, tearful, moving, unfamiliar, archetypal, growthful. For me it means the full embrace of life—the savouring of all its subtle tastes. (p. 34)

A Concluding Metaphor

Stuttering is a highly complex problem in which behaviors, thoughts, and feelings are interwoven and interactive. Not a disease or a syndrome, it arises in individual ways and, as has been discussed, is strikingly influenced in its development by the changing interactions of self and family in the preschool years.

Once developed and locked in with the automaticity of language and speech production, it is more like a place than a disorder—a place where the person is lost and afraid, tangled in an underbrush of struggle, unable to see the way out or even know where or how to start looking for it. Ironically, there are almost as many paths leading out of this forest as there are leading into it. First, people who stutter have to find out where they are. Then they have to learn that struggling only creates more entanglements. Once they understand and accept this, they find they are on their metaphorical way out.

The speech clinician with academic knowledge of stuttering and experience with people who stutter has a general map of this area, but it lacks detail. The person who stutters has a very detailed map of where he or she is at the moment, but too often denial has made the map itself difficult to see, as if the page was dim and blurred. Together, client and clinician can fill in the details and adjust the focus through a particular kind of conversation, changing each other's understanding of this place and finding a path to freedom.

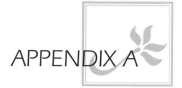

APPENDIX A

Guidelines for Practice in Stuttering Treatment

Special Interest Division on Fluency and Fluency Disorders
of the American Speech-Language-Hearing Association[1]

Those guidelines are an official statement of the American Speech-Language-Hearing Association (ASHA). They are guidelines for practice in stuttering treatment but are not official standards of the association. They were developed by members of the Steering Committee of ASHA's Special Interest Division on Fluency and Fluency Disorders (Division 4): C. W. Starkweather, Kenneth O. St. Louis, Gordon Blood, Theodore Peters, Janice Westbrook, Hugo Gregory, Eugene Cooper, and Charles Healey, under the guidance of Crystal Cooper, vice president for professional practices. Lyn Goldberg provided support from the national office. The Steering Committee acknowledges the assistance of Diane L. Eger, vice president for professional practices from 1991 to 1993.

I. Introduction

The document that follows was developed by the Special Interest Division in Fluency and Fluency Disorders (SID4) of ASHA in response to the affiliates' belief that the field lacked standards for the treatment of stuttering. It was felt, too, that the parallel move toward specialization made it necessary to define more clearly the role of non-specialists. At the same time, the ASHA document Preferred Practice Patterns for the Professions of Speech-Language Pathology and

[1]Reprinted, with changes, by permission of the American Speech-Language-Hearing Association.

Audiology (ASHA Supplement No. 11, March 1993) was published but addressed only Fluency Assessment and only in the most general terms. The failure of this document to address the treatment of fluency disorders left a gap to be filled.

It should be noted that the Steering Committee felt that the state of knowledge in several key areas—treatment efficacy and the measurement of stuttering specifically—was not developed well enough to allow the promulgation of "standards." It was decided to provide "guidelines," which would be less prescriptive.

Another issue concerned the base of knowledge used to determine whether a goal is desirable or a practice appropriate to achieve a goal. The SC felt that a set of criteria for determining guidelines based entirely on empirical evidence would be too restrictive. Some treatment practices may be quite useful even though their efficacy has not yet been determined empirically. The committee felt that both common practice and published data should be considered.

Finally, the SC does not take a position on stuttering theory or on a philosophy of treatment. Instead, the draft is written on what is hoped to be an agreed upon set of goals, and procedures that are used to achieve them.

II. General Guidelines for Practice

A. Timing and Duration of Treatment

There is considerable variation in the timing and duration of therapy sessions and in the total duration of therapy. Some residential programs treat clients very intensively, 6 or more hours each day for a number of weeks. Private clinicians may see clients one, two, or three times a week for a longer period of time. In the schools and hospitals, the timing and duration of sessions is restrained by overriding schedules. Intensive treatment may be expected to achieve more rapid change, but the intensive treatment alters the client's daily activity more extensively, creating a barrier to transfer that the clinician considers in planning therapy activities. Nonintensive treatment, on the other hand, disrupts the client's everyday life far less, but it may achieve change so slowly that the client becomes discouraged. Clinicians who see clients less frequently can sequence therapy activity for early success or provide for other motivational activities that will keep the client interested in continuing treatment.

B. The Setting of Treatment

Clients are seen in a wide variety of settings. Some programs are residential, providing treatment, usually intensive, in a setting removed from the client's everyday life. Others treat the client in the community where he or she lives. Both residential and nonresidential treatment programs provide activities for effective transfer of new behaviors to the ordinary social situations of everyday life. Transfer can be achieved through carefully sequenced, monitored practice in real-life social situations. Programs that treat the client only in a limited setting and do not provide for monitored practice of newly learned behaviors in natural settings fall outside the guidelines of good practice. There are a number of ways to monitor a client's practice: (a) direct observation, in which the clinician is present during the practice session, (b) interviews with the client after practice sessions, and (c) listening, with the client, to audiotape recordings of practice sessions. In each case, monitoring should include opportunities for the clinician to discuss the practice session with the client so as to increase understanding, and opportunities to provide immediate feedback on the client's performance. Listening to audiotape recordings that are submitted by mail and responded to with written comments from the clinician falls outside the guidelines of good practice, if it is the only method of transfer. It should be recognized, however, that there are circumstances—when a client lives in a remote area, for example—where it may be impossible to provide service that is within the guidelines. The best practice, in these circumstances, is to make sure that both client and clinicians are aware of any necessary limitations on treatment.

There is also variation in the duration of individual sessions. In general, clinicians plan sessions so that they are long enough to accomplish some stated objective, but not so long as to lose the client's attention through fatigue or boredom. The client's age and his or her ability to attend are taken into consideration in determining the duration of sessions.

C. Duration of Treatment

The total duration of therapy is an important variable of practice. Clinicians want to be sure that therapy lasts long enough for effective change, but they do not want to continue to provide treatment when there is no longer any further benefit. Our field is in the process of researching the variables that impact treatment duration, but we cannot yet say with certainty what these variables are. It seems clear that more intensive treatment produces more rapid change than nonintensive treatment (Prins, 1970). It also seems likely, but not yet demonstrated, that the complexity of a client's problem may influence the duration of treatment. People who stutter in a way that is unusually complex behaviorally, or who have other coexisting problems or disorders, are likely to require considerable time in treatment. Those who are cognitively impaired, or who cannot attend easily, for example, would be expected to take longer in therapy. Also, the presence of a coexisting language or articulation disorder, or a psychoemotional disturbance, can lengthen treatment.

A client's personal level of motivation and commitment to the therapy process will also influence the duration of therapy. School-age, adolescent, and adult stutterers require longer durations of treatment than preschool children. In spite of the uncertainty that remains in this area, clinicians try to provide to clients and their families some sense of how long therapy may take, including the processes of maintenance and follow-up.

D. Complexity of Treatment

Stuttering is typically a complex problem. It may begin somewhat simply, but it usually, and sometimes quickly, becomes complex by the reactions, defensive behaviors, and coping strategies of the person who stutters and by the reactions of significant others in the listening environment. Furthermore, in older children and adults, the communicative difficulties that stuttering creates present barriers to social, educational, and vocational life that can greatly complicate the problem. In some cases, there can be serious emotional disturbance, such as depression or sociopathic behavior. These complexities create issues that clinicians help their clients deal with through therapy and referral. Stuttering therapies that do not address the complete problem in whatever complexity it presents are not within the guidelines of good practice.

E. The Cost of Treatment

As independent professionals, clinicians working with stutterers have the responsibility of setting their own fees. In doing so, they consider a number of factors. People who stutter sometimes seek help with an intense longing for relief, and in some cases feel quite desperate. Clinicians, in setting their fees, do not exploit these feelings. In addition, the client's desire for help can be increased through statements by the clinician implying that the treatment is highly effective. The prohibition in the Code of Ethics of ASHA against misrepresentation in public statements has particular relevance for stuttering therapy. When clinicians make public statements about their own treatment programs, they are appropriately cautious about its effectiveness. It would seem well outside the guidelines of good practice for a clinician to make a public statement that a new technique could solve every stutterer's problem, and then charge far more than is the usual practice. The setting in which treatment takes place may also be a factor in determining the cost of treatment. Treatment in the schools is free (or at least paid for indirectly), and treatment offered in hospital settings must follow fee guidelines determined by the hospital. In some settings, or under some special circumstances, there may be an inherent limitation on the quality of service offered, suggesting that it would be appropriate to set the fees below the going rate. For example, some university training programs, but not all, feel that the quality of their service is altered by the fact that they have to meet training standards. A program that feels that their training mission detracts from their therapy could appropriately decide to reduce its fees.

Typically, the amount of time the clinician spends in face-to-face contact with the client is the main yardstick by which the value of therapy is determined. Telephone contact, tape recordings, paper, and electronic mail contact also have value, although not many clinicians charge for these services. The value of therapy for people who stutter lies in the supportive nature of the client–clinician relationship and in the clinician's ability to hear and see the stutterer's behavior and respond to it in a way that helps the client learn to talk in a more effective way.

III. Attributes of Clinicians Who Work with People Who Stutter

It is desirable for clinicians to have certain personal attitudes and qualities and a fund of certain information. The following list is an expanded version of the Texas Speech and Hearing Association Fluency Task Force's list of "Personal Clinician Competencies":

A. Personal Attributes

1. Is interested in and committed to the treatment of people with fluency disorders.

2. Is willing to develop as much knowledge and skill as possible related to diagnosis and treatment of stuttering and keeps abreast of current developments.

3. Is willing to refer clients when the need for more assistance is necessary.

4. Is willing to take an active role in the profession to know about specific services that are available both locally and nationally to clients who stutter.

5. Has good problem-solving skills and uses them when things do not go according to plan in evaluation and treatment.

6. Is flexible in thinking and planning.

B. Learned Attributes

7. Has a general understanding of the literature relative to the etiology and development of stuttering.

8. Has an adequate level of knowledge of the phenomenology of stuttering, particularly with regard to those phenomena that influence therapeutic practice, such as, for example, episodic variation, clustering, paradoxical intention, adaptation and consistency, spontaneous recovery, fluency enhancement, arousal effects, etc.

9. Has a general understanding of the literature on normal and language-based (dys)fluency, rate, prosody, rhythm, and effort and the development of these speech characteristics and has the skill to gain new information from the literature as new findings are incorporated into it.

10. Has a view of stuttering that is focused enough to provide planning of therapy but broad and adjustable enough to accommodate research findings and theoretical perspectives.

11. Has an understanding and appreciation of the possible relations between a person's normal and abnormal speech behavior on the one hand and their beliefs, upbringing, and cultural background on the other.

12. Has an understanding and appreciation of the basic processes of dynamic therapeutic interaction, such as transference, denial, grief, victimization.

13. Can communicate relevant ideas about stuttering to clients and their parents.

14. Has a general working knowledge of psychopathology.

15. Has a general working knowledge of cognitive and behavioral learning theory.

In addition, the specialist in fluency should meet the guidelines listed below.

IV. Specific Guidelines for Practice—Goals, Processes, and Competencies

This section contains three parts. First, a list of goals, appropriate to the treatment of fluency disorders, is described. The criterion for including a goal in this list is that they be acceptable and desirable goals for speech–language pathologists to try to reach with fluency-disordered clients. These goals follow from the nature of fluency disorders, and it is expected that few will disagree with the choice of goals. Indeed, narrow peer review revealed a very broad consensus on the goals.

The philosophy of treatment that a clinician believes in will, of course, strongly determine which goals are considered most important. This list is intended to include all goals that are considered appropriate by all philosophies of treatment currently held by speech–language pathologists who treat people who stutter. The order of goals presented in this document does not reflect their order of importance.

It is recognized that certain goals may be desirable for (some) clients to reach but are nevertheless outside the scope of practice for most speech–language pathologists, for example, psychotherapeutic goals unrelated to fluency, or parenting issues unrelated to a child's fluency.

The second part lists processes that are useful for achieving specific goals. The inclusion of processes in this list in no way mandates their use by clinicians. Some clinicians will rely exclusively on a few processes; others will combine many different processes. The list is an attempt to set down processes that are in widespread use by speech–language pathologists who treat stuttering.

The criteria for selecting processes combines empirical knowledge, theory, and common practice. For example, one goal is a reduction in the frequency of stuttering behaviors. Processes that have been shown empirically to reduce stuttering behaviors in a lasting way, for example, slowed parental speech rate for young stuttering children, have consequently been included. Another process, for example, instrumental extinction, might be included for more theoretical reasons. In some cases either the empirical or the theoretical support is weak, and this weakness is pointed out in the document.

The third part identifies competencies—skills and knowledge—that clinicians can use in order to engage in the processes identified in Part 2. The criteria for inclusion in this list of competencies is simply logical. If the modification of cognitive structures that make it difficult for a client to think about his or her speech in a productive way is a desirable goal, then cognitive restructuring is a useful process, and a competency in that technique is useful for clinicians to have. It is understood that not all clinicians will have all competencies, although it is expected that clinicians will continue to augment their current competencies through continuing education.

A. Assessment

Desirable goals in the assessment of fluency disorders:

Assessment Goals

1. Obtain a speech sample that is as representative as possible of the client's speech in everyday use.

2. Obtain a sample of the client's speech under circumstances that are constant from one client to the next.

3. Generate, from obtained speech samples and incidental observations, quantitative and qualitative descriptions of the client's fluent and dysfluent speech behavior that can be related where applicable to vocal tract physiology, and that are communicable to other interested professionals.

4. Obtain information about variables that affect the client's fluency level and apply this to therapy planning.

5. Obtain information about a client's early social, physical, behavioral, and speech development, including information about variables that might be related to the origin of the disorder or its course of development, and apply this information to therapy planning.

6. Obtain information about variables that might influence therapeutic outcome and/or the prognosis for treatment and apply this to therapy planning.

7. Obtain information about other communicative problems or disorders that may or may not be related to fluency.

8. Generate descriptions of the results of assessment that are communicable to other professional and lay persons.

B. Processes for Achieving the Goals of Assessment

Processes for Achieving Assessment Goal 1— Achieving a Representative Sample

1. Observation and recording of the client's speech during an interview with the clinician about the client's stuttering problem.

2. Surreptitious observation and recording of the client talking to a relative or friend in the waiting room prior to meeting with the clinician.

3. Observation and recording of a child playing with parents after instructions to the parents to play with the child as you normally would at home (Family Play Session).

4. Tape recordings made by the client of conversations he or she has held during daily activities at work, home, or anywhere.

Processes for Achieving Assessment Goal 2— A Speech Sample from a Constant Setting

1. Observation and recording of the client's speech in response to being asked to describe a standard stimulus picture.

2. Observation and recording of the client's speech while he or she reads a standard passage aloud.

3. Observation and recording of the client's speech while the client plays a "barrier game" with the clinician, or, preferably, with a third party.

4. Observation and recording of the client's speech during a structured interview, in which the clinician asks the same question of each client by referring to an interview form.

5. Observation and recording of the client's speech while he or she performs a specific speech task, such as describing a job, a favorite activity, or a school subject.

Processes for Achieving Assessment Goal 3—Quantitative and Qualitative Description of the Client's Fluency Level

1. Administering any of a variety of published tests of fluency, stuttering severity, attitudes toward stuttering and speech, self-efficacy as a speaker, situational fears, and avoidance behavior.

2. Administering any of a variety of systematic protocols for coding speech sample(s) so as to reflect the categories of dysfluency, and the extent of fluency or nonfluency, and the presence and type of secondary behaviors.

3. Transcribing a speech sample verbatim in such a way as to accurately reflect all fluent and nonfluent speech behavior.

4. Identifying and counting the frequency of primary and secondary stuttering behaviors.

5. Measuring the duration of discontinuous and continuous speech elements.

6. Measuring speech rate (syllables per second with pauses included) and articulatory rate (syllables per second with pauses excluded).

7. Observation and recording behavioral and/or physiological measurements of oral, laryngeal, and respiratory behavior so as to relate specifically identified stuttering behaviors to possible vocal tract events and to assess the capacity for fluent speech production.

8. Describing qualitatively any of the nonmeasurable aspects of fluency, such as apparent level of muscular tension, emotional reactivity to speech or stuttering behaviors, coping behaviors, nonverbal aspects of stuttering behavior, or anom-

alies of social interaction such as poor eye contact, generalized low muscle tonus, poor body posture, etc.

Processes for Achieving Assessment Goal 4— Assessing Variables That Affect Fluency

1. Developing and systematically testing hypotheses about variables that might affect fluency level, for example, talking
   slowly to a stuttering child to see if a measurable improvement in fluency can be obtained.

2. Interviewing the client or the client's parents about social circumstances, words, listeners, sentence types, speech sounds,
   that improve or exacerbate fluency.

3. Playing videotapes or audiotapes of parent–child interactions
   to the parents of a child who presents a potential or actual
   fluency disorder.

4. Conducting a variety of brief trial therapy procedures, such
   as delayed auditory feedback, whispering, rate modification,
   etc.

Processes for Achieving Assessment Goal 5— Getting and Using a Developmental History

1. Developing questionnaires or other written materials (e.g.,
   fluency autobiography) designed to obtain potentially relevant background information.

2. Interviewing the client, the client's parents, or others about
   developmental milestones of motor control, social–emotional
   behavior, speech and language, and cognitive level.

Processes for Achieving Assessment Goal 6— Getting and Using Prognostic Information and Information That Will Optimize Therapy Planning

1. Administering or reading reports of others who have administered formal test of intelligence, attitudes, motivation, comprehension, ability to take direction, or prognostic indicators.

2. Informal tests and observations related to intelligence, attitudes, motivation, comprehension, ability to take direction, or
   other prognostic indicators.

Processes for Achieving Assessment Goal 7— Getting and Using Information About Coexisting Problems

1. Administering tests or reading reports of others who have administered formal tests of language, voice, articulation, psycho-emotional function, learning disability, cognitive level, or auditory or visual deficits and using this information to plan for therapy and to provide prognostic information.

2. Making informal observations of language, voice, articulation, psycho-emotional function, learning disability, cognitive level, or auditory or visual deficits and using this information to plan for therapy and to provide prognostic information.

Processes for Achieving Assessment Goal 8— Communicating the Results of Assessment

1. Writing reports of assessment processes designed to be read by physicians, psychologists, and other nonspeech–language pathology professionals.

2. Writing comprehensive reports of assessment processes designed to be read by the current or subsequent clinicians.

3. Reporting the results of assessment processes, formally or informally, to the client and/or the client's parents.

C. Clinician Competencies Related to Assessment

1. Can differentiate between a child's normally disfluent speech, language-based disfluency, the speech of a child at risk for stuttering, and the speech of a child who has already begun to stutter.

2. Can distinguish cluttered from stuttered speech and understands the potential relations between these two disorders.

3. Can relate the findings of language, articulation, voice, and hearing tests to the development of stuttering.

4. Can obtain a thorough case history from an adult client or the parents of a child client.

5. Can obtain a useful speech sample and evaluate it for stuttering severity both informally by subjective impression and for

mally by calculating relevant measures such as the frequency of dysfluency, duration of dysfluency, speaking rate, etc.

6. Is familiar with the available diagnostic tests for stuttering that serve to objectify aspects of the client's communication pattern (secondary features, avoidance patterns, attitudes, etc.) that may not be readily observed.

7. Is able to identify, and measure where feasible, environmental variables (i.e., aspects such as time pressure, emotional reactions, interruptions, nonverbal behavior, demand speech, or the speech of significant others) that may be related to the onset, development, and maintenance of stuttering and to fluctuations in the severity of stuttering.

8. Can identify dysfluencies by type (prolongation, repetition, etc.) and, in addition, can describe qualitatively the fluency of a person's speech.

9. Can relate, to the extent possible, what stuttered speech sounds like to the vocal tract behavior that is producing it (for example, recognizing the subtle acoustic cues that signal vocal straining).

10. Can, in appropriate consultation with the client or parents, construct a treatment program, based on the results of comprehensive testing, on the client's personal emotional and attitudinal development, and on past therapeutic history, that fits the unique needs of each client's problem(s).

11. Can administer predetermined programs in a diagnostic way so that decisions with regard to branching and repeating of parts of the program reflect the unique needs of each client's problem(s).

12. Can explain clearly to clients or their parents what treatment options, including the various types of speech therapy, medication, devices, self-help groups, and other forms of therapy are available, why they may or may not be appropriate to a specific case, and what outcomes can be expected from each, based on knowledge of the available literature.

D. Management

Desirable goals in the management of fluency disorders:

Management Goals

1. Reduce the frequency with which stuttering behaviors occur without increasing use of other behaviors that are not a part of normal speech production.

2. Reduce the severity, duration, and abnormality of stuttering behaviors until they are or resemble normal speech discontinuities.

3. Reduce the use of defensive behaviors. Note that when clients use avoidance behaviors that are successful (in that they avoid stuttering behavior) they will appear to have made progress toward Management Goal 1, but in fact will have done so by including some additional, and abnormal, behavior. For example, a client who is able to change words so as to avoid saying a word that he or she will stutter on will have a reduced frequency of stuttering behavior, but he or she will also have an increased frequency of cognitive behaviors involved in the search for and retrieval of substitute words.

4. Remove or reduce learning, or other processes serving to create, exacerbate, or maintain stuttering behaviors. In children, this might entail modification of the child's parents' behavior so as to reduce maladaptive reactions to the child's stuttering behavior. In adults it might include teaching the client how to change his or her listeners' behavior. In some cases, there may be reinforcement for stuttering, such as excuses for failure, or getting attention that is otherwise not forthcoming. In other cases, denial may prevent an adult from perceiving the extent to which stuttering impacts his or her life.

5. Help the person who stutters make therapeutic (e.g., adaptive) decisions about how to handle speech and social situations in everyday living. This includes such things as helping the client learn how to respond to people who try to talk for him or her, or helping the client learn not to use behaviors that avoid, rather than confront, specific social situations such as using the telephone, ordering in a restaurant, or helping the client learn that changing words costs something in personal self-esteem. This also includes teaching the client how to politely influence listeners' behavior so that the client's fluency can be improved.

6. Increase the frequency of social activity and speaking. Clients who have adopted reticence as a strategy to deal with stuttering will need help in regaining a normal amount of social speech.

7. Reduce attitudes, beliefs, and thought processes that interfere with fluent speech production or that hinder the achievement of other therapeutic goals. In some adults this might involve modifying their attitude toward very brief stuttering behaviors so as to prevent stuttering from returning at a later date. Similarly, certain attitudes toward fluency and dysfluency, or beliefs about these behaviors, can serve processes that maintain stuttering behaviors, for example, perfectionistic fluency, abhorrence of normal dysfluency, rigidity in speech behavior. Some clients may have attitudes toward themselves that serve to exacerbate or maintain stuttering behaviors, for example, low self-esteem, lack of confidence, or feelings of worthlessness.

8. Reduce emotional reactions to specific stimuli when these impact negatively on stuttering behavior or on attempts to modify stuttering behavior. For example, fear of specific social situations, word fears, a sense of intimidation by specific categories of listeners, a sense of helplessness or fear of specific speech tasks, such as answering the telephone, asking questions in class, etc., or a fear of the embarrassment of stuttering in public. This should not be confused with the reduction of defensive behavior, which is one kind of reaction to these fears. Both fear reduction and defensive behavior reduction can be appropriate.

9. Where necessary, seek helpful combinations and sequences of therapies and treatments, including referral, for problems other than stuttering that may accompany the fluency disorder, for example, cluttering, learning disability, language/phonological disorder, voice disorder, psycho-emotional disturbance.

10. Provide information and guidance to clients, families, and other significant persons about the nature of stuttering, normal fluency and dysfluency, and the course of treatment and prognosis for recovery. In addition, help clients and parents understand the nature of past treatment and the availability and possible utility of other treatment options, including other forms of therapy, therapeutic devices, and self-help groups.

E. Processes for Achieving the Goals of Management

It is not the intention of this document to assert that all processes should be used with all clients. A process for reducing excitement is useful only with a client whose fluency is adversely influenced by excitement. For each client, clinicians choose a set of appropriate goals, based on a careful evaluation of the client. Having established what are appropriate goals for a client, a selection of processes to achieve these goals is made. At times during therapy, both goals and processes should be reevaluated, and after therapy, it is likewise appropriate to review the selection of goals and processes and evaluate them with regard to the outcome of treatment.

Note that processes are not exactly the same as techniques. There might be several techniques for engaging in a particular process. For example, one process mentioned below is "Identify reinforcers for stuttering." A clinician could engage in this process by interviewing the client and asking what happens after he or she stutters, by spending some time with the client, observing him or her in real speaking situations, or by interviewing people who know the client well, such as parents, siblings, partners, etc. Each of these techniques would or could result in the identification of reinforcers that are contingent on stuttering behavior.

Note that referral and consultation are processes that may be used to achieve goals.

Processes for Achieving Management Goal 1— Reducing the Frequency of Stuttering Behaviors

1. Fluency-shaping approach

   a. Slowed rate of speech movements

      • Typically taught in stages of speed (e.g., Rate I, Rate II, and Slow-Normal Rate)

   b. Easy onset of voicing

      • Slow inhalation

      • Soft but true voice changing to full voice before vowel initiation

      • Practice in order to shorten the time taken up by the onset of voicing period

    c. Blending, or continuous voicing

    d. Light articulatory contacts

    e. Smooth, slow speech movements

    f. Use of computer-assisted feedback to train clients in fluency-producing coordinated speech production movements

2. Vocal control therapy approach

    a. Better vocal tone, breath support, full resonance, efficient and relaxed voice, adequate loudness

    b. Typically accompanied by systematic desensitization

3. Contingency management

    a. Combined reinforcement for fluent speech and mild, non-aversive punishment for stuttering behaviors

    b. Successive approximation (shaping) toward fluent speech

    c. Practice in a systematically sequenced series of steps from where fluent speech is easiest to achieve toward where fluency is more difficult to achieve, for example, through gradually increasing the length and complexity of utterance, or through a hierarchy of feared social situations

    d. Use of fluency-enhancement, in the clinic, or via a wearable device, may be a useful way to initially establish the behavior

    e. Use of computer-assisted devices to ensure rapid and consistent feedback

    f. Systematically administered reinforcement for more natural-sounding speech

4. Reduction of speech-associated anxiety

    a. Systematic desensitization to social situations

    b. Desensitization to the experience of stuttering (confrontation)

    c. Pseudostuttering (voluntary stuttering, or faking)

    d. With children, through counseling parents, reduction or removal of as many anxiety-producing events as possible

5. Reduction of speech-associated excitement

    a. With children, through counseling parents, reduction of as many exciting events as practical and reasonable

6. In prevention, training parents to speak more slowly but with normal intonation, timing, and stress patterns

7. In prevention, training parents to talk less often, and with simpler language, to interrupt less often, and to ask fewer questions requiring long complex answers

Processes for Achieving Management Goal 2—Reducing the Abnormality, Severity, or Duration of Stuttering Behaviors

1. Dysfluency shaping

    a. Help the client learn ways to be dysfluent in a more normal way

    b. Remove, through modeling and practice, one behavior at a time until dysfluencies are normal in type

2. Muscle tension reduction

    a. Reduction of oral and vocal muscular tension during speech

      • Slowed rate and rate control

      • Direct suggestion to reduce muscle tension in specific parts of the vocal tract

      • Referrals for the possible use of medication to achieve muscle relaxation

      • Attitude modification via techniques described below

3. Repair treatment

    a. Teach client the various types of speech sounds and how they are fluently produced

    b. Teach client the types of stuttering behaviors used by client

    c. Teach client types of repairs—ways of changing from the stuttered to the nonstuttered type of production

    d. Practicing repairs in different environments

e. Work on one or two specific sounds or sound categories at a time

4. Stuttering modification sequence

a. Post-block modification, or cancellation

b. In-block modification, or pull-out

c. Pre-block modification, or preparatory set

5. Counterconditioning techniques

a. Associating stuttering with pleasant events, for example, "reinforcement" for stuttering, or tag game, etc.

b. Voluntary stuttering

6. Confrontational (nonavoidance) techniques

a. Discussion with the client of specific behaviors, the circumstances under which they occurred, and the variables that may have influenced them

b. Watching with clients audio- or videotapes of the client while speaking and discussing specific behaviors and reactions with him

Processes for Achieving Management Goal 3— Reducing Defensive Behaviors

1. Extinction of defensive behavior

a. For secondary (avoidance) behavior:

- Direct instructions to stop performing the secondary behavior accompanied by an alternative to stuttering behavior, for example, in-block modification (pull-outs), or slowed speech, or monitored vocalization

- Punishment (time-out, response cost or other nonaversive punishment only) accompanied by an alternative to stuttering behavior

b. For primary (escape) behavior, that is, struggled dysfluency

- Stuttering modification sequence of post-block, in-block, pre-block modification

- Modeling stuttering that is easy and free of struggle, then reinforcing the client for dysfluency that is less struggled

- Direct suggestions, accompanied by cueing and reminders

- Discussions about the clients stuttering pattern, approaching feared situations, to toughen attitudes toward stuttering

2. In prevention, training parents in the relaxed production of occasional dysfluencies that are normal for their child's age

Processes for Achieving Management Goal 4—Removing Processes That May Be Maintaining Stuttering Behaviors

1. Instrumental (operant) conditioning

   a. Identify reinforcers for stuttering

   b. Remove conditions in the environment, including the client's "internal environment" that are reinforcing stuttering or defensive behavior

2. Defensive counterconditioning

   a. Identify aversive consequences for stuttering

   b. Identify stimuli, or constellations of stimuli (situations) associated with or predictive of aversive consequences, as in a hierarchy of speech situations

   c. Identify behaviors that terminate or avoid the aversive consequences

   d. Provide experiences for the client in which the conditioned stimuli occur, but the avoidance behaviors are *not* performed and no aversive consequences follow

   e. Help client learn how to handle pressure situations while still using newly learned fluency skills

3. Vicarious conditioning

   a. Identify speech models who are (a) reinforced for stuttering, (b) who avoid stuttering or try to avoid stuttering (i.e., use defensive behavior), or (c) who demonstrate negative emotional reactions to dysfluency

b. Counsel, train, or modify the behavior of these models so as to remove or reduce the occurrence of vicarious conditioning

4. Environmental manipulation

Alter the client's environment, external or internal, so as to remove any conditioning process that is exacerbating or maintaining stuttering behavior

- By counseling significant others

- By counseling the client

- By providing for experiences that will alter attitudes or beliefs of that result in deleterious conditioning processes

Processes for Achieving Management Goal 5— Helping Clients Learn How to Make Therapeutic Decisions about Everyday Speaking Situations

1. Identification of specific decisions about social behavior that may affect fluency, for example, deciding to let a colleague answer the phone even though the client is closer to it

2. Counseling, including sensitive explanations about how decisions based on defensive reactions serve to increase fear and decrease self-confidence

3. Identify, with the client's help, attainable behavioral goals for more therapeutic decision making

4. Plan activities that will provide opportunities for the decisions

5. Reinforce client for making decisions that are more conducive to speaking fluently and with confidence

6. Help clients foresee the natural consequences of their decisions to use or not to use learned treatment techniques in day-to-day activities

7. Attendance in a support group with other people who stutter

Processes for Achieving Management Goal 6— Increasing Social Activity and Speaking Behavior

1. Provide reinforcement for entering speech situations previously feared

2. Encouragement and reinforcement for talking more often and in a wider variety of situations, structured hierarchically from least to most stressful or intimidating

3. Encourage client to participate in a self-help group

4. Use of a fluency-enhancing device to make possible social activity that would otherwise be too intimidating for the client

Processes for Achieving Management Goal 7— Improving Self-Esteem or Revising a Perfectionistic Attitude Toward Speech

1. Counsel the client so as to provide for successful experiences of any kind

2. Counsel the client so as to provide for successful speech experiences

3. Validation of the client as a person and speaker

   a. Listen to the client and demonstrate appreciation of the client as a person

   b. Listen to the client and validate aspects of speech that are unrelated to fluency, through expressed appreciation for aspects of the client's speech that are normal or superior, for example, voice quality, expressiveness, word choice, articulation

   c. Listen to the client and validate his or her fluency, where appropriate, by expressed appreciation for stuttering behaviors that are less struggled or less abnormal

   d. Transfer of similar listening skills to client (self-listening)

4. Provide for increased attention from significant others

5. Help client attain better identification of self through support-group or other activities

6. Provide for increased tolerance of failings through counseling, modeling

7. Positive self-talk and affirmation training

Processes for Achieving Management Goal 8— Reducing Negative Reactions to Stuttering and Social Situations That Have Included Stuttering in the Past

1. Confrontational desensitization to stuttering events

a. Talking about stuttering with the client in an objective way

b. Have the client learn, through self-demonstration, that his/her speech improves when he/she "gives permission to stutter" or stutters on purpose

c. Stuttering on purpose in the clinical setting

d. Stuttering on purpose in real situations

e. Keep a record of situations in which the client has stuttered on purpose or allowed him/herself to stutter

2. Desensitize to anxiety-provoking speech situations

   a. Traditional systematic desensitization

      • Constructing a hierarchy of feared words, listeners, and situations

      • Inducing a physically and emotionally relaxed state

      • Imagining feared situations while in a relaxed state

      • Imagining oneself talking to feared listeners while in a relaxed state

      • Imagining oneself producing feared words while in a relaxed state

      • Imagining oneself stuttering while in a relaxed state

      • Testing the effects of these experiences in real situations

   b. In vivo systematic desensitization

      • Constructing a hierarchy of feared words, listeners, and situations

      • Systematically talking in real life situations, starting with the easiest elements in the hierarchy, and gradually increasing the level of difficulty. A fluency-enhancing device may provide a place to begin this process, although it will be important to wean the client from the device so as not to create a dependency on it

Processes for Achieving Management Goal 9— Dealing with Coexisting Problems

1. Referral to other professionals with regard to psychoemotional or learning disability problems

2. Team treatment with other speech–language pathologists so as to work simultaneously on language, phonological, or voice problems

3. Sequencing therapy so as to deal with one problem first, then with the other. Usually this means postponing work on language, voice, or articulation until fluency is under control, but sometimes it means postponing work on fluency until some progress is made on the other problem, for example, improved intelligibility

4. Designing treatment plans that deal simultaneously with stuttering and coexisting problems

Processes for Achieving Management Goal 10— Providing Information to Significant Others

1. Direct counseling of parents, spouses, siblings, etc.

2. Bibliotherapy for parents, spouses, physicians, psychologists, etc.

3. Use of audio- and videotape to present to clients and the parents of clients examples of specific behaviors and reactions

4. Provide information about other therapeutic approaches, therapeutic devices, self-help and consumer advocate groups

5. Provide information about third-party payment options

F. Clinician Competencies Related to Management

1. Is familiar with the appropriate goals of therapy and the processes for achieving them and can engage these processes, choosing techniques that are best for the client, and administer them with an attitude that balances the goal of normal speech with a tolerance for abnormal speech.

2. Has flexibility in choosing and changing the level of difficulty of tasks based on fluency level of the client.

3. Can teach clients to produce vocal tract behaviors that result in normal sounding speech production.

4. Has sufficient counseling skills so as to interact with clients of all ages and develop a reasonable set of expectations in the client.

5. Has a thorough understanding of, and knows how to put into practice, the principles of conditioning and learning so

as to achieve a successful and appropriate modification of speech behavior.

6. Understands the relations between stuttering and other related disorders of fluency, such as cluttering, neurogenic, and psychogenic stuttering, as well as disorders of language, articulation, learning, etc., and can with flexibility identify sequences and combinations of treatment options that are helpful to the client.

7. Understands the dimensions of normal fluency and the relation of normal fluency to the speech situations and is able to work toward normal speech, with an awareness of the compromises among effort, fluency, and natural-sounding communication.

8. Understands that some stuttering behaviors may be reactions to other stuttering behaviors and knows how to plan treatment so as to account for this.

9. Can evaluate available therapy programs with regard to therapeutic application for a wide variety of clients.

10. Is able to decide, based on objective progress, motivational level, and cost in time and money, when it is appropriate to terminate therapy.

11. Is aware of the continuous nature of fluency and can identify subtle changes in speech or other behaviors related to therapeutic change and explain their importance to the client.

12. Can explain stuttering and therapy for stuttering to lay persons, such as day-care workers, teachers, baby-sitters, grandparents, etc., who may influence the life of stuttering children.

13. Knows how to develop a plan for assessing objectively the efficacy of treatment during therapy in an ongoing way.

14. Can recognize problems that are treated by professionals other than speech–language pathologists and can guide a client to acceptance of an appropriate referral.

G. Transfer and Maintenance

Desirable goals in the transfer and maintenance of acquired fluency behaviors.

Transfer and Maintenance Goals

1. Generalization of the behavioral changes learned in the treatment setting to speech situations in the client's everyday life.

2. A sense of committed interest and self-reliance on the part of clients in managing their own speech behavior, balanced against an awareness of the need for occasional help (professional or otherwise) as needed.

3. Ability on the client's part at recognizing the earliest signs of returning emotional reactions and/or stuttering behaviors and knowledge and skill for dealing with this problem.

4. In parents, knowledge and skills needed to facilitate their child's further development of fluency.

H. Processes for Achieving Transfer and Maintenance Goals

Processes for Achieving Transfer and Maintenance Goal 1— Generalization of Behavior to External Settings

1. Variation of speech use within the treatment setting.

2. Role playing of social interactions while using new behaviors.

3. Hierarchically structured practice in the client's everyday life, monitored by the clinician via tape recordings and/or interviews.

4. Continued practice in the treatment setting.

5. Use of self-help and support groups.

Process for Achieving Transfer and Maintenance Goal 2— Self-Reliance and Commitment

1. Counseling the client to assist him or her in taking over the process of decision making in treatment.

2. Providing exercises for the client designed to increase skills at self-evaluation and self-therapy planning.

3. Gradually reducing the clinician's input in making decisions about treatment.

4. Gradually decreasing the frequency of therapeutic contact between clinician and client.

5. Use of self-help and support groups.

Processes for Achieving Transfer and Maintenance Goal 3— Self-Monitored Maintenance

1. Practice at self-listening and identification of stuttering behaviors, even brief or barely noticeable ones.

2. Counseling and training in the modification of brief and barely noticeable stuttering behaviors.

3. Counseling and training at recognizing changes in client's attitude, specifically increasing tendency to avoid speech situations and/or stuttering.

4. Use of self-help and support groups.

Processes for Achieving Transfer and Maintenance Goal 4— Parent Facilitation of Child's Fluency Development

1. Counseling and training families in recognition of subtle signs of returning struggle.

2. Desensitization and empowerment of parents so as to reduce anxious reactions to signs of returning struggle behavior.

3. Training parents and other family members in skills useful in providing a fluency-enhancing atmosphere.

4. Use of family support groups.

I. Clinician Competencies Related to Transfer and Maintenance

1. Is aware of the principles of stimulus generalization and response transfer.

2. Has knowledge of, and can implement a variety of procedures to achieve transfer and maintenance of behavior changes achieved in the clinical setting.

3. Can, through guidance and counseling, help clients develop an attitude toward maintenance that includes an

understanding of their own responsibility for their speech yet permits occasional booster session (e.g., the dental model) and that tolerates failure yet appreciates success.

4. Can help the client develop an awareness of the subtler forms of (returning) abnormality and know how to deal with them in a variety of ways, such as the use of home practice, graded hierarchical practice in social situations, and support groups.

5. Knows how to counsel parents regarding changes they can make at home that will facilitate their child's fluency development or encourage the generalization of gains made in treatment.

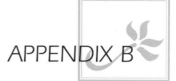

APPENDIX B

A Story for Group Telling to Preschool Children at Risk for Stuttering

"Boo" Goodnight to Halloween

by Tracy Harrison

Every Halloween, after all the candy is collected and all the children have gone to bed, the Halloween ghosts come out to "boo" goodnight to Halloween. When the clock strikes midnight all the ghosts fly around in the night sky and "boo" goodnight to Halloween.

Some ghosts "boo" loud, some ghosts "boo" soft, some ghosts "boo" long and some ghosts "boo" short. It's the ghosts' favorite night of the year.

On one Halloween many years ago one ghost almost didn't get to say goodnight to Halloween. This is what happened . . .

One Halloween just before midnight, all the ghosts were knocking on each others' doors and rushing around to get ready to "boo" goodnight to Halloween.

Knock, knock, knock. "Hurry up, it's almost time to 'boo' goodnight to Halloween," one ghost said to another.

Peter the ghost was flying high in the sky with all the other ghosts when he noticed his best friend Sammy the ghost was not around.

"Where is Sammy?" asked Peter ghost.

"I don't know," said Lisa ghost.

"I don't know either," said Bobby ghost.

"I will go and find him," said Peter ghost.

"Hurry up," said Lisa ghost. "It's almost midnight."

Peter quickly flew to Sammy's house and knocked at the door. Sammy opened the door.

"Sammy, c'mon. It's almost midnight, and we have to 'boo' goodnight to Halloween."

"I'm not 'booing' goodnight to Halloween," Sammy ghost said.

"Why?" asked Peter.

"Because sometimes when I 'boo, boo, boo' I get stuck."

"Sometimes you get stuck?" asked Peter.

"Yes, sometimes I get stuck."

"Well, that's okay, Sammy, every ghost gets stuck sometimes when they 'boo.'"

"Really?" Sammy asked.

"Really. I get stuck sometimes too," Peter said.

"Well, in that case, let's hurry before it's too late," Sammy said.

Sammy and Peter ghost then flew as fast as they could into the night sky so they could catch up with the other ghosts in time to "'Boo' goodnight to Halloween!"

The End

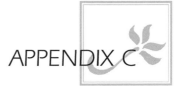

APPENDIX C

Resources for the Person Who Stutters

Aaron's Associates
6114 Waterway
Garland, TX 75043
USA

**The American
Speech–Language–Hearing
Association**
10801 Rockville Pike
Rockville, MD 20852
USA

**Association Belges des Bègues
et Ex-Bègues**
Rue des Peupliers 10
B-7730 Estaimpus
Belgium

**Association de Bègues de
France (A.B.F.)**
Rue de Romaineville 26
F-931000 Montreuil
France

**Association Française des
Bègues (AFB)**
Rue du Général de Gaulle 60
F-68240 Kaysersberg
France

**Associazione "La Lingua
Amara"**
Casella Postale 189
I-56100 Pisa Pl
Italy

BEVOS
Fruithoflaan 101
B-2600 Berchem
Belgium

The Birch Tree Foundation
457 Old Farm Road
Wyncote, PA 19095
USA

The British Stammerer's Association
St. Margaret's House
21 Old Ford Road
Bethnal Green
London E2 9PL
UK

Bundesvereinigung Stotterer-Selbsthilfe
Geroenswall 113
D-50670 Köln
Germany

The Canadian Association for People Who Stutter
228 Galoway Road, Suite 309
Scarborough, Ontario M1E 5G6
Canada

Compulsive Stutterers Anonymous
c/o Susan Reed
506 Lynn Avenue
Sycamore, IL 60178
USA

Demosthenes
Schmidtné Bálas Eszter
H-1118 Budapest
Rezeda u. 9
Hungary

Estonian Association for People Who Stutter (EAPS)
c/o Andres Loorand
Tartumaa
Alatskivi vald EE-2415
Estonia

The European League of Stuttering Associations
Geroenswall 113
D-50670 Köln
Germany

Foreniging for Stammere i Danmark
c/o DSI
Kløverprisvej 10B
DK-2650 Hvidovre
Denmark

The International Fluency Association
Box 870242
Tuscaloosa, AL 35487
USA

José Nadales Sánchez
c/o Hortezuela, 21
E-29150 Almoga (Málaga)
Spain

Lithuanian Stuttering Club
Malonioji 5
2004 Vilnius
Lithuania

MALBJÖRG
ph. 10043
IS-130 Reykjavik
Iceland

Marina Llobera O'Brien
Despacho: Palma Rehabilitacion
Vasco de Gama, 11
(esq. Andrea Doria)
E-07014 Palma de Mallorca
Spain

**The National Council on
Stuttering**
c/o Connie Dugan
Counseling Center, M/C 333
University of Illinois at Chicago
1200 West Harrison Street
Chicago, IL
USA

The National Stuttering Project
5100 E. La Palma Avenue,
Suite 208
Anaheim Hills, CA 92807
USA
800/364-1677

**Nederlandse Stottervereniging
"Demosthenes"**
Postbus 119
NL-3500 AC Utrecht
The Netherlands

**Norsk Interesseorganisasjon for
Stammen (NIFS)**
PO Box 114 - Kjelsaas
N-0411 Oslo
Norway

**Österreich-Selbsthilfe-Initiative
für Stottern (ÖSIS)**
Brixner Strasse 3
A-6020 Innsbruck
Austria

Polski Zwiazek
Jakajacych sie (PZJ)
ul. Dunajewskiego 6/21
PL-31-133 Kraków
Poland

Schwätzen ouni Angscht
4, place Boltgen
L-4044 Esch-sur-Alzette
Luxemburg

**Speakeasy International
Foundation, Inc.**
233 Concord Drive
Paramus, NJ 07652
USA

**The Stuttering Foundation of
America**
1539 Klingle Street, NW
Washington, DC
USA
800/967-7700

**The Stuttering Information
Centre of Denmark**
Emdrupvej 101
DK-2400 Copenhagen, NV.
Denmark

The Stuttering Resource Foundation
123 Oxford Road
New Rochelle, NY 10802
USA

Suomen änkyttäjien yhdistys ry (SÄY) Finska Stammares
Förening rf (FSF)
Box 60
FIN-0031 Helsinki
Finland

The Swedish Stammering Association
Sveriges Stamningsföreningars
Riksförbund (SSR)
Box 9514
S-102 74 Stockholm
Sweden

Vereinigung für Stotternde und Angehörige
Bleiken
CH-3775 Lenk i./S
Switzerland

V.Z.W.-BEST
Belangengroep Stotterars
H. Moeremanslaan 40
B-1700 Dilbeek
Belgium

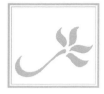

References

Adams, M. R. (1975). Letter to the editor. *Journal of Speech and Hearing Research, 40*, 136.

Adams, M. R. (1990). The demands and capacities model I: Theoretical elaborations. *Journal of Fluency Disorders, 15*, 135–142.

Adams, M. R., & Ramig, P. (1980). Vocal characteristics of stutterers and normal speakers during choral reading, *Journal of Speech and Hearing Research, 23*, 457–465.

Ahlbach, J. (1995). *To say what is ours.* San Francisco: The National Stuttering Project.

Americans with Disabilities Act of 1990, 42 U.S.C. §12101 *et seq.*

Amsel, A., & Ward, J. (1954). Motivational properties of frustration: II. Frustration drive stimulus and frustration reduction in selective learning. *Journal of Experimental Psychology, 48*, 37–47.

Amster, B. (1984). *The rate of speech in normal preschool children.* Unpublished doctoral dissertation, Temple University, Philadelphia, PA.

Amster, B. (1989, November). *Case studies in language overstimulation and stuttering.* Convention address at the annual meeting of the American Speech-Language-Hearing Association, St. Louis, MO.

Amster, B. (1995). Perfectionism and stuttering. In C. W. Starkweather, H. F. M. Peters (Eds.), *Proceedings of the First World Congress on Fluency Disorders, Munich, Germany, 1994* (pp. 540–543). Nijmegen, The Netherlands: University of Nijmegen Press.

Anderson, H., & Goolishian, H. (1988). Human systems as linguistic systems: Preliminary and evolving ideas about the implications for clinical theory. *Family Process, 27*, 371–393.

Andrews, G., Craig, A., Feyer, A-M., Hoddinott, S., Howie, P., & Neilson, M. (1983). Stuttering: A review of research findings and theories circa 1982. *Journal of Speech and Hearing Disorders, 48,* 226–246.

Andrews, G., & Harris, M. (1964). *The syndrome of stuttering.* London: Heinemann.

Armson, J. (1991). *A study of laryngeal muscle activity during stuttering episodes: Searching for an invariant physiological correlate.* Unpublished doctoral dissertation, Temple University, Philadelphia, PA.

Bandura, A. (1969). *Principles of behavior modification.* New York: Holt.

Beattie, M. (1990a). *Codependents' guide to the twelve steps: How to find the right program for you and apply each of the twelve steps to your needs.* Englewood Cliffs, NJ: Prentice-Hall.

Beattie, M. (1990b). *The language of letting go: Daily meditations for codependents.* New York: Harper-Collins.

Bedore, L. M., & Leonard, L. B. (1995). Prosodic and syntactic bootstrapping and their clinical applications. *American Journal of Speech–Language Pathology, 4,* 66–72.

Berry, M. F. (1938). Developmental history of stuttering children. *Journal of Pediatrics, 12,* 209–217.

Bloodstein, O. (1960). The development of stuttering I. Changes in nine basic features. *Journal of Speech and Hearing Disorders, 25,* 219–237.

Bloodstein, O. (1987). *The handbook of stuttering* (4th ed.). Chicago: National Easter Seal Society.

Bobrick, B. (1995). *Knotted tongues.* New York: Simon and Schuster.

Borden, G. (1982, November). *Initiation versus execution time during manual and oral counting by stutterers.* Convention address at the annual meeting of the American Speech-Language-Hearing Association, Toronto.

Brady, J. P. (1995). The role of pharmacology in the treatment of stuttering. In C. W. Starkweather & H. F. M. Peters (Eds.), *Proceedings of the First World Congress on Fluency Disorders, Munich, Germany, 1994* (pp. 508–510). Nijmegen, The Netherlands: University of Nijmegen Press.

Brauth, S. E., Hall, W. S., & Dooling, R. J. (Eds.). (1991). *Plasticity of development.* Cambridge, MA: MIT Press.

Breitenfeldt, D., & Lorenz, D. (1995). A therapy demonstration of the Successful Management Program. In C. W. Starkweather & H. F. M.

Peters (Eds.), *Proceedings of the First World Congress on Fluency Disorders, Munich, Germany, 1994* (pp. 309–312). Nijmegen, The Netherlands: University of Nijmegen Press.

Brutten, G. J., & Shoemaker, D. J. (1967). *The modification of stuttering.* Englewood Cliffs, NJ: Prentice-Hall.

Caruso, A., Abbs, J., & Gracco, V. (1988). Kinematic analysis of multiple movement during speech in stutterers. *Brain, 111,* 439–455.

Caruso, A., Conture, E., & Coulton, R. (1988). Selected temporal parameters of coordination associated with stuttering in children, *Journal of Fluency Disorders, 12,* 57–82.

Cecconi, C. P., Hood, S. B., & Tucker, R. K. (1977). Influence of reading level difficulty on the disfluencies of normal children. *Journal of Speech and Hearing Research, 20,* 475–484.

Darley, F. (1955). The relationship of parental attitudes and adjustments to the development of stuttering. In W. Johnson & R. R. Leutenegger (Eds.), *Stuttering in children and adults.* Minneapolis: University of Minnesota Press.

De Nil, L., & Brutten, G. (1988). *Homorganic and heteroganic consonant clusters in stutterers' and nonstutterers' fluent speech.* Paper presented at the annual meeting of the American Speech-Language-Hearing Association, Boston.

Farber, S. (1981). *Identical twins reared apart: A reanalysis.* New York: Basic Books.

Ford, S. C., & Luper, H. L. (1975, November). *Aerodynamic, phonatory, and labial EMG patterns during fluent and stuttered speech.* Convention address at the annual meeting of the American Speech-Language-Hearing Association, Washington, DC.

Franken, M. C., Peters, H. F. M., & Tettero, C. M. (1989). Evaluation of the Dutch version of Webster's Precision Fluency Shaping Program for stutterers. *Logopedie en Foniatrie, Jaargang 61* (11), 343–345.

Franken, M. C., Konst, E., Boves, L., & Rietveld, T. (1995). The effect of intonation contours on the acceptability of treated stutterers' speech. In C. W. Starkweather & H. F. M. Peters (Eds.), *Proceedings of the First World Congress on Fluency Disorders, Munich, Germany, 1994* (pp. 432–435). Nijmegen, The Netherlands: University of Nijmegen Press.

Fransella, F., & Beech, H. R. (1965). An experimental analysis of the effect of rhythm on the speech of stutterers. *Behavior Research and Therapy, 3,* 195–201.

Freeman, F. (1975). Letter to the editor. *Journal of Speech and Hearing Research,* *40,* 137.

Freeman, F., & Ushijima, T. (1978). Laryngeal muscle activity during stuttering. *Journal of Speech and Hearing Research, 21,* 538–562.

Garber, S. F., & Martin, R. R. (1977). Effects of noise on increased vocal intensity and stuttering. *Journal of Speech and Hearing Research, 20,* 233–240.

Goldman-Eisler, F. (1961). The continuity of speech utterance: Its determinants and its significance. *Language and Speech, 4,* 220–231.

Gordon, P., Luper, H., & Peterson, H. (1986). The effects of syntactic complexity on the occurrence of disfluencies in 5-year-old children. *Journal of Fluency Disorders, 11,* 151–164.

Gordon, P., & Peterson, H. (1982, November). *Analysis of preschool dysfluency for sentence-imitation and sentence-modeling.* Convention address at the annual meeting of the American Speech-Language-Hearing Association, Toronto.

Hegde, M. N., & Hartman, D. (1979a). Factors affecting judgments of fluency: I. Interjections. *Journal of Fluency Disorders, 4,* 1–12.

Hegde, M. N., & Hartman, D. (1979b). Factors affecting judgments of fluency: II. Word repetitions. *Journal of Fluency Disorders, 4,* 13–22.

Helm, N. A., Butler, R. B., & Canter, G. J. (1980). Neurogenic acquired stuttering. *Journal of Fluency Disorders, 5,* 269–279.

Hill, H. (1954). An experimental study of disorganization of speech and manual responses in normal subjects. *Journal of Speech and Hearing Research, 19,* 295–305.

Hofstadter, D. (1979). *Gödel, Escher, Bach: An eternal golden braid.* New York: Random.

Hood, S. (Ed.). (1974). *To the stutterer.* Memphis, TN: Speech Foundation of America.

Howie, P. M. (1981). Concordance for stuttering in monozygotic and dizygotic twin pairs. *Journal of Speech and Hearing Research, 24,* 317–321.

Hurst, M., & Cooper, E. (1983). Employer attitudes toward stuttering. *Journal of Fluency Disorders, 8,* 1–12.

Ingham, R. (1984). *Stuttering and behavior therapy: Current status and experimental foundations.* San Diego, CA: College-Hill.

Ingham, R., & Cordes, A. (1992). Interclinic differences in stuttering-event counts. *Journal of Fluency Disorders, 17,* 171–176.

Johnson, W. (1955). A study of the onset and development of stuttering. In W. Johnson & R. R. Leutenegger (Eds.), *Stuttering in children and adults*. Minneapolis: University of Minnesota Press.

Johnson, W., & Associates. (1959). *The onset of stuttering*. Minneapolis: University of Minnesota Press.

Kalinowski, J., Armson, J., & Stuart, A. (1995). Effects of alterations in auditory feedback on stuttering frequency during fast and normal speech rates. In C. W. Starkweather & H. F. M. Peters (Eds.), *Proceedings of the First World Congress on Fluency Disorders, Munich, Germany, 1994* (pp. 51–55). Nijmegen, The Netherlands: University of Nijmegen Press.

Kalinowski, J., Noble, S., Armson, J., & Stuart, A. (1994). Pretreatment and posttreatment speech naturalness ratings of adults with mild and severe stuttering. *American Journal of Speech–Language Pathology: A Journal of Clinical Practice, 3,* 61–66.

Kidd, K. (1980). Genetic models of stuttering. *Journal of Fluency Disorders, 5,* 187–201.

Kimble, G. (1961). *Hilgard and Marquis' conditioning and learning* (2nd ed.). New York: Appleton-Century-Crofts.

Kinsbourne, M., & Hicks, R. E. (1978). Mapping cerebral functional space: Competition and collaboration in human performance. In M. Kinsbourne (Ed.), *Asymmetrical function of the brain* (pp. 234–247). Cambridge, MA: Cambridge University Press.

Klich, R., & May, G. (1982). Spectrographic study of vowels in stutterers: Fluent speech, *Journal of Speech and Hearing Research, 25,* 364–370.

Kline, M. L., & Starkweather, C. W. (1979, November). *Receptive and expressive language performance in young stutterers.* Convention address at the annual meeting of the American Speech-Language-Hearing Association, Atlanta.

Kloth, S. A. M., Janssen, P., Kraaimaat, F. W., & Brutten, G. (1995). Speech-motor and linguistic skills of young stutterers prior to onset. *Journal of Fluency Disorders, 20,* 157–170.

Kowal, S., O'Connell, D. C., & Sabin, E. F. (1975). Development of temporal patterning and vocal hesitations in spontaneous narratives. *Journal of Psycholinguistic Research, 4,* 195–207.

Krashen, S. (1973). Lateralization, language learning, and the critical period: Some new evidence. *Language Learning, 23,* 63–74.

Laris, J. (1994). Here's looking at you. In J. Ahlbach (Ed.), *To say what is ours* (pp. 89–90). San Francisco: National Stuttering Project.

Levelt, W. J. M. (1989). *Speaking: From intention to articulation.* Cambridge, MA: MIT Press.

Longhurst, T. M., & Siegel, G. M. (1973). Effects of communication failure on speaker–listener behavior. *Journal of Speech and Hearing Disorders, 16,* 128–140.

Ludlow, C. (1996). *Neurological correlates of stuttering.* Paper presented at the annual leadership conference of the Special Interest Division on Fluency, Monterey, CA.

Lutz, K. C., & Mallard, A. R. (1986). Disfluencies and rate of speech in young adult nonstutterers. *Journal of Fluency Disorders, 11,* 307–316.

Malecot, A., Johnston, R., & Kizziar, P.-A. (1972). Syllabic rate and utterance length in French. *Phonetica, 26,* 235–251.

Martin, R., Haroldson, S., & Triden, K. (1984). Stuttering and speech naturalness. *Journal of Fluency Disorders, 49,* 53–58.

Meltzer, A. (1992). Horn stuttering. *Journal of Fluency Disorders, 17,* 257–264.

Merits-Patterson, R., & Reed, C. (1981). Disfluencies in the speech of language-disordered children. *Journal of Speech and Hearing Research, 46,* 55–58.

Meyers-Fosnot, S. (1992, April 23). *Management of stuttering in young children.* American Speech-Language-Hearing Association teleconference.

Montgomery, B. M., & Fitch, J. L. (1988). The prevalence of stuttering in the hearing-impaired population. *Journal of Speech and Hearing Disorders, 53,* 131–135.

Milisen, R., & Johnson, W. (1936). A comparative study of stutterers, former stutterers, and normal speakers whose handedness has been changed. *Archives of Speech, 1,* 61–86.

Parry, W. (1994). *Understanding and controlling stuttering.* San Francisco: National Stuttering Project.

Perkins, W. (1971). *Speech pathology: An applied behavioral science.* St. Louis, MO: Mosby.

Perkins, W., Kent, R., & Curlee, R. (1991). A theory of neuropsycholinguistic function in stuttering. *Journal of Speech and Hearing Research, 34,* 734–752.

Peters, H. F. M., & Hulstijn, W. (1984). Stuttering and anxiety: The difference between stutterers and nonstutterers in verbal apprehension and physiologic arousal during the anticipation of speech and nonspeech tasks. *Journal of Fluency Disorders, 9,* 67–84.

Peters, H. F. M., Hulstijn, W., & Starkweather, C. W. (1989). Acoustic and physiological reaction times of stutterers and nonstutterers. *Journal of Speech and Hearing Research, 32,* 668–680.

Peters, H. F. M., Hulstijn, W., & van Lieshout, P. (1995). Towards a Nijmegen speech motor test. In C. W. Starkweather & H. F. M. Peters (Eds.), *Stuttering: Proceedings of the First World Congress on Fluency Disorders, Munich, Germany, 1994* (pp. 15–18). Nijmegen, The Netherlands: University of Nijmegen Press.

Peters, H. F. M., & Starkweather, C. W. (1990a). The development of stuttering throughout life. *Journal of Fluency Disorders, 15,* 107–114.

Peters, H. F. M., & Starkweather, C. W. (1990b). The interaction between speech motor coordination and language processes in the development of stuttering: Hypotheses and suggestions for research. *Journal of Fluency Disorders, 15,* 115–125.

Peters, T., & Guitar, B. (1991). *Stuttering: An integrated approach to its nature and treatment.* Baltimore: Williams & Wilkins.

Prins, D. (1970). Improvement and regression in stutterers following short-term intensive therapy. *Journal of Speech and Hearing Disorders, 35,* 123–135.

Prins, D. (1991). Theories of stuttering as event and disorder: Implications for speech production processes. In *Proceedings of the Conference on Fluency and Speech Motor Control, Nijmegen, The Netherlands, 1990* (pp. 291–306). Amsterdam/New York: Elsevier.

Preus, A. (1981). *Identifying subgroups of stutterers.* Oslo: Universitetsforlaget.

Ramig, P. (1993). The impact of self-help groups on persons who stutter: A call for research. *Journal of Fluency Disorders, 18,* 351–362.

Reed, S. (n.d.). *Compulsive Stutterers Anonymous: 12 steps to recovery.* Park Ridge, IL: Compulsive Stutterers Anonymous.

Roman, K. G. (1959). Handwriting and speech. *Logos, 2,* 29–39.

Roth, C. R., Aronson, A. E., & Davis, L. J., Jr. (1989). Clinical studies in psychogenic stuttering of adult onset. *Journal of Speech and Hearing Disorders, 54,* 634–646.

Schaef, A. W. (1992). *Beyond therapy, beyond science.* New York: HarperCollins.

Schwartz, M. F. (1974). The core of the stuttering block. *Journal of Speech and Hearing Disorders, 39,* 169–177.

Schwartz, M. F. (1976). *Stuttering solved.* New York: McGraw-Hill.

Scripture, E. W. (1909). Penmanship and stuttering. *Journal of the American Medical Association, 52,* 1480–1481.

Shames, G., & Florance, C. (1980). *Stutter-free speech: A goal for therapy.* Columbus, OH: Merrill.

Sheehan, J. G. (1970). *Stuttering: Research and theory.* New York: Harper.

Sheehan, J. G. (1974). Stuttering behaviors: A phonetic analysis. *Journal of Communication Disorders, 7,* 193–212.

Sheehan, J. G., & Martyn, M. M. (1970). Spontaneous recovery from stuttering. *Journal of Speech and Hearing Research, 9,* 279–289.

Shields, D. (1986). *Dead languages.* New York: Harper & Row.

Smith, A. (1989). Neural drive to muscles in stuttering. *Journal of Speech and Hearing Research, 32,* 252–264.

Smith, A. (1995). Muscle activity in stuttering. In C. W. Starkweather & H. F. M. Peters (Eds.), *Proceedings of the First World Congress on Fluency Disorders, Munich, Germany, 1994* (pp. 39–42). Nijmegen, The Netherlands: University of Nijmegen Press.

Soderberg, G. (1966). The relations of stuttering to word length and word frequency. *Journal of Speech and Hearing Research, 9,* 584–589.

Stager, S., & Siren, K. (1995). A comparison of botulinum toxin injection and clomipramine treatments. In C. W. Starkweather & H. F. M. Peters (Eds.), *Proceedings of the First World Congress on Fluency Disorders, Munich, Germany, 1994* (p. 515). Nijmegen, The Netherlands: University of Nijmegen Press.

Starkweather, C. W. (1982). *Stuttering and laryngeal behavior: A review* (ASHA Monograph No. 21). Rockville, MD: American Speech-Language-Hearing Association.

Starkweather, C. W. (1987). *Fluency and stuttering.* Englewood Cliffs, NJ: Prentice-Hall.

Starkweather, C. W. (1991). Stuttering: The motor-language interface. In H. Peters, W. Hulstijn, & C. Starkweather (Eds.), *Speech motor control and fluency. Proceedings of the Conference on Fluency and Speech Motor Control, Nijmegen, The Netherlands, 1990* (pp. 220–225). Amsterdam/New York: Elsevier Science Pub. Co.

Starkweather, C. W. (1994). *Current practices in stuttering therapy.* Paper presented at the annual leadership conference of the Special Interest Division on Fluency, Hilton Head, South Carolina.

Starkweather, C. W. (1995a). The electronic self-help group. In C. W. Starkweather & H. F. M. Peters (Eds.), *Stuttering: Proceedings of the First World Congress on Fluency Disorders, Munich, Germany, 1994* (pp. 499–503). Nijmegen, The Netherlands: University of Nijmegen Press.

Starkweather, C. W. (1995b). A simple theory of stuttering. *Journal of Fluency Disorders, 20,* 91–116.

Starkweather, C. W. (1996). The role of learning processes in the development of stuttering. In R. Curlee & G. Siegel (Eds.), *Nature and treatment of stuttering: New directions* (2nd ed.). Boston: Allyn & Bacon.

Starkweather, C. W., & Bishop, J. (1994). *Required practicum hours in fluency: A survey of training supervisors.* Report to the Council on Professional Standards, ASHA.

Starkweather, C. W., Blood, G., Peters, T., St. Louis, K., & Westbrook, J. (1993). Standards of practice in stuttering therapy. *Newsletter of the Fluency Special Interest Division of ASHA.*

Starkweather, C. W., Blood, G., St. Louis, K., Peters, T., & Westbrook, J. (1995). *Guidelines for the practice of stuttering therapy.* Rockville, MD: American Speech-Language-Hearing Association.

Starkweather, C. W., Gottwald, S. R., & Halfond, M. H. (1990). *Stuttering prevention: A clinical method.* Englewood Cliffs, NJ: Prentice-Hall.

Starkweather, C. W., & Myers, M. (1979). The duration of subsegments within the intervocalic interval in stutterers and nonstutterers. *Journal of Fluency Disorders, 4,* 205–214.

Starkweather, C. W., & Peters, H. F. M. (Eds.). (1995). *Proceedings of the First World Congress on Fluency Disorders, Munich, Germany, 1994.* Nijmegen, The Netherlands: University of Nijmegen Press.

Stephenson-Opsal, D., & Bernstein-Ratner, N. (1988). Maternal speech rate modification and childhood stuttering. *Journal of Fluency Disorders, 13,* 49–56.

St. Louis, K., & Daly, D. (1995). Cluttering: Past, present and future. In C. W. Starkweather & H. F. M. Peters (Eds.), *Proceedings of the First World Congress on Fluency Disorders, Munich, Germany, 1994* (pp. 659–662). Nijmegen, The Netherlands: University of Nijmegen Press.

St. Louis, K., & Sielen, R. (1994a, November). *Person-first labels: Public impressions and experiences.* Poster session presented at the annual convention of the American Speech-Language-Hearing Association, New Orleans.

St. Louis, K., & Sielen, R. (1994b, November). *Person-first labels: Public views of appropriate use.* Poster session presented at the annual convention of the America Speech-Language-Hearing Association, New Orleans.

Tiffany, W. R. (1980). The effects of syllable structure on diadochokinetic and reading rates. *Journal of Speech and Hearing Research, 23*, 894–908.

Tuck, A. (1979). An alaryngeal stutterer: A case history. *Journal of Fluency Disorders, 4*, 239–243.

Van Lancker, D., Canter, G., & Terbeek, D. (1981). Disambiguation of ditrophic sentences: Acoustic and phonetic cues. *Journal of Speech and Hearing Research, 24*, 330–335.

van Lieshout, P. H. H. M., Peters, H. F. M., Starkweather, C. W., & Hulstijn, W. (1993). Physiological differences between stutterers and nonstutterers in perceptually fluent speech: EMG amplitude and duration. *Journal of Speech and Hearing Research, 36*, 55–63.

van Lieshout, P. H. H. M., Starkweather, C. W., Hulstijn, W., & Peters, H. F. M. (1995). Effects of linguistic correlates of stuttering on EMG activity in nonstuttering speakers. *Journal of Speech and Hearing Research, 38*, 360–372.

Van Riper, C. (1963). *Speech correction: Principles and methods* (4th ed.). Englewood Cliffs, NJ: Prentice-Hall.

Van Riper, C. (1973). *The treatment of stuttering.* Englewood Cliffs, NJ: Prentice-Hall.

Van Riper, C. (1982). *The nature of stuttering* (2nd ed.). Englewood Cliffs, NJ: Prentice-Hall.

Walker, C., & Black, J. W. (1950). *The intrinsic intensity of oral phrases* (Joint Project Report No. 2). Pensacola, FL: Naval Air Station, U.S. Naval School of Aviation Medicine.

Wall, M. J., & Myers, F. L. (1995). *Clinical management of childhood stuttering* (2nd ed.). Austin, TX: PRO-ED.

Webster, R. L. (1972). *An operant response shaping program for the establishment of fluency in stutterers: Final report.* Hollins College, VA: Hollins College.

White, P. A., & Collins, S. R. C. (1984). Stereotype formation by inference: A possible explanation for the "stutterer" stereotype. *Journal of Speech and Hearing Research, 27*, 567–570.

Wingate, M. E. (1964). A standard definition of stuttering. *Journal of Speech and Hearing Disorders, 29*, 484–489.

Wingate, M. E. (1971). The fear of stuttering. *Asha, 13*, 3–5.

Wingate, M. E. (1976). *Stuttering: Theory and treatment.* New York: Irvington.

Wingate, M. E. (1981). Questionnaire study of laryngectomee stutterers. *Journal of Fluency Disorders, 6*, 273–281.

Yairi, E. (1982). Longitudinal studies of disfluencies in two-year-old children. *Journal of Speech and Hearing Research, 25,* 155–160.

Yairi, E. (1992, September). *Research of efficacy treatment in stuttering: Preschool children.* Workshop, National Institutes of Health, Bethesda, MD.

Young, M. (1984). Identification of stuttering and stutterers. In R. Curlee & W. Perkins (Eds.), *Nature and treatment of stuttering: New directions* (pp. 13–30). San Diego: College-Hill.

Zimmermann, G. (1980). Stuttering: A disorder of movement. *Journal of Speech and Hearing Research, 23,* 122–136.

Zinker, J. (1977). *Creative process in Gestalt therapy.* New York: Random.

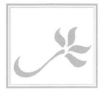

Index

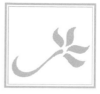

About the Authors

Janet Givens-Ackerman, who has stuttered since the age of 6, is now in recovery from stuttering. She is a co-director of the Birch Tree Foundation with experience in 12-step recovery programs and Gestalt experiential therapy dating back to 1990. Ms. Givens-Ackerman holds a BS from NYU and an MA from Kent State University, both in sociology. She currently works for the University of Pennsylvania in their development and alumni relations efforts.

C. Woodruff Starkweather received his BA in English from Hamilton College and his PhD in speech pathology from Southern Illinois University. He has worked exclusively with people who stutter since 1965 and is currently the president of the International Fluency Association. The author of seven books and over 50 chapters and articles on stuttering, Dr. Starkweather developed the demands and capacities model of stuttering development and founded the stuttering prevention center at Temple University. He is the principal author of the *Guidelines for Stuttering Therapy* of the American Speech-Language-Hearing Association and co-director of the Birch Tree Foundation.

Notes

Notes

Notes